FIT FOR THE MASTER

Glorifying God in a Healthy Body

FIT FOR THE MASTER

Glorifying God in a Healthy Body

John Lehman

First Edition: 2015

Printed in the United States of America

ISBN: 978-0-9899532-9-0

Published by www.greatwriting.org

Cover designed by Greg Warner

Our Christianity should affect every area of our lives—including our health and fitness. In *Fit for the Master* John not only shows you how to be fit—he also tells you why, as a Christian, you should be fit. Read this book and then go live this book.

Jeremy McMorris, Lead Pastor, Liberty Baptist Church, Dalhart, TX

The complexity of creation with its purpose and the complexity of the human body with its purpose meet in an easy-to-read and easy-to-follow book on fitness for everyone. *Fit for the Master* offers excellent and safe advice on how and why to get fit.

Roger Bachour, PT, TPI certified, Accelerated Physical Therapy

Fit for the Master is a wonderful resource full of practical advice and insights into living a well-balanced life. John Lehman not only writes about these ideas—he practically lives them out every day! If you desire to live a more effective and efficient life, then I would strongly recommend this book.

James Whitaker, Men's Soccer Coach and Assistant Athletic Director, Columbia International University

In *Fit for the Master*, Lehman offers a compelling and scripturally based discussion of two topics—Christian faith and physical fitness—that, at first glance may seem unrelated, but which are actually closely connected. This book provides readers with clear, understandable, and practical guidance on how and why to begin or improve a fitness and nutrition regimen. It is a valuable resource to Christians who seek to apply their faith in every facet of their lives, and I commend it to you.

Miles Coleman, Corporate Attorney, Nelson Mullins Riley & Scarborough, LLP; Ironman triathlete, ultra-marathoner, and CrossFit coach

Physical discipline is a necessity for a Christian to be effective. John lays out the "why" and the "how" in this encouraging and challenging book.

Aaron Iles, Catskill Mountain 100 km course record holder, NCCAA D1 Cross Country All-America, Quoted in Trail Runner Magazine, Sub 24 hr finish of Pine Creek Challenge 100 miler

Against the backdrop of a self-consumed society that pushes weight-loss tricks, fad diets, and elaborate fitness routines, *Fit for the Master* applies biblical wisdom and scientific evidence while making commonsense recommendations for physical exercise, nutrition, and sleep. Whether you are a seasoned veteran or a rookie, I hope you will find—as I have found over the miles with John Lehman—the spiritual encouragement and essentials to improve or develop a healthy lifestyle.

Russell Davis, Captain, United States Marine Corp; USSF and NISOA referee and runner

Purpose

"This book is intended to encourage everyone to be fit for the Master's use. God created us, and therefore we should be as functional as possible, so bringing Him glory while being able to lead more efficient and effective lives."

It has been a wonderful blessing to apply the principles that are within this book. Early in my life I simply trusted and applied them, and as I've grown older, have benefited from the results.

.

John Lehman

www.fitforthemaster.fit

Dedication

I would like to dedicate this book to the athletes with whom I've been associated as coach or training partner. Great joy has been mine through the relationships I've forged through exercise! That alone has been wonderful, but the benefits of the exercise have been a tremendous help to me through these years. It has been through this that the idea of this book was formulated.

I often think of Hebrews 10:24 which states that we are to "consider how to stir up one another to love and good works." You have all helped me to be better in fitness, which has helped me in all aspects of life.

As is always noted, there is nothing good in me, except what God has created and entrusted. I could never pursue fitness, or anything else for that matter, without God's gracious and helpful watch care over my life. He's the One who receives any glory for any good done in and through me!

Acknowledgements

I extend great appreciation to the following:

Greg Warner, who designed the book cover: Thank you for your efforts to get just the right design and detail.

Greg and Emily Warner, who drew and illustrated the graphics and examples for the stretches and exercises: Thanks for making sure everything portrayed was what was intended.

Jonathan Wooster, who filmed and edited my promotional video for the book: Your expertise, in yet another discipline, helped in this presentation.

Brent Heidorn, who reviewed and suggested material which assisted with specificity due to his expertise: Your work helped me refine and define, and I appreciate your desire to sharpen me.

Jim Holmes, who has worked tirelessly to format and "shape" this book into its final product: None of this would have come together without your oversight. You have helped me by gently directing, helpfully guiding, and continually encouraging my every step.

Suzie, who has encouraged me through yet another writing project: "Many women have done excellently, but you surpass them all" (Proverbs 31:29).

Chapter Contents

A Note on Gender

To avoid being slavish and using he or she, him or her, and his or hers, etc., the use of pronouns in this text has been deliberately varied. Also, please keep in mind that terms such as "mankind" and "man" are intended to be understood in a gender-inclusive way!

Foreword

I t brings me great pleasure to have the opportunity to support my good friend, John Lehman, in his recent accomplishments with his new book, *Fit for the Master*. As I think of John, many fine qualities come to mind, including committed man of God; responsible and loving husband and father of four grown children; long-time pastor and Bible scholar; and fitness and sports enthusiast.

John demonstrates the epitome of health, physical activity, and continuous energy, while remaining actively involved in so many different pursuits. As a fitness fanatic myself, I have participated with John in many athletic endeavors, including cycling, swimming, basketball, tennis, racquetball, softball, weight training, and, most notably, hundreds of hours pounding the pavement and trails. John has a true passion for physical fitness, and effectively uses his similar interests with others as opportunities to grow, mentor, and share the gospel. John has been one of my mentors for several years. He consistently discusses his faith and relationship with God, but also engages in conversations related to exercise physiology, intervals, nutrition, marathon training, and more.

The content in this book challenges all of us to reflect upon our relationship with God our Creator, and realize that we are fearfully and wonderfully made (Psalm 139:14). Using the framework of 1 Corinthians 6:19-20, John comprehensively explains many basic and complicated components for living healthy, physically active lives. This book is a must-read for anyone interested in beginning, maintaining, or improving his or her level of physical fitness, while also exploring the biblical reasons we should seek godliness through exercise.

Brent Heidorn, Ph.D.
Assistant Dean for Research and Assessment
Associate Professor in Health and Physical Education
University of West Georgia in Carrollton, GA

1

Glorious Creator;
Wonderful Creation

Thinking about your place in God's universe

See, this alone I found, that God made man upright, but they have sought out many schemes.

(Ecclesiastes 7:29)

God is the God of physical creation. He made a tangible, physical universe, a universe composed of stuff. It may well be said that, to God, matter matters. He, the Author of life, created the heavens and the earth. He then created the sun, moon, stars, plants, animals, and man. Man was the only created being formed in God's image.

God, Himself a Spirit, intended from the beginning of time to communicate with and have a relationship with the physical, flesh-and-blood people He had created. That was the initial and major reason He brought the world into being. God's simple statement was: "It [is] good." In Revelation 4:11 it is written, "Worthy are you, our Lord and God, to receive glory and honor and power, for you created all things, and by your will they existed and were created."

Man was created so that he could bring glory to God and have a relationship with Him. Scripture specifically records that man was made in the image and likeness of God (see Genesis 1:26). If sin had never entered the world, it appears that man would have lived forever, and without the catastrophic consequences of eating the fruit of the tree of the knowledge of good and evil, from which he had expressly been forbidden to eat.

Because the wages of sin is death, the whole of the created realm was affected by the disobedience of Adam and Eve. Sin entered the world. And with sin came several consequences: separation from God, pain in childbirth, intensive frustration in work, sickness and disease, and—ultimately—physical death. Death is the separation of the body from the soul.

At the very beginning, everything was good; in fact, everything was perfect—that is, until the ruin that came about by the fall. This brought in its wake the consequences of deterioration and death.

From Ruin to Redemption

However, God did not leave it at that. In one of the best known passages in the Bible, it is written: "For God so loved the world, that he gave his only Son, that whoever believes in him should not perish but have eternal life. For God did not send his Son into the world to condemn the world, but in order that the world might be saved through him" (John 3:16, 17).

Titus 2:11-14 states "For the grace of God has appeared, bringing salvation for all people, training us to renounce ungodliness and worldly passions, and to live self-controlled, upright, and godly lives in the present age, waiting for our blessed hope, the appearing of the glory of our great God and Savior Jesus Christ, who gave himself for us to redeem us from all lawlessness and to purify for himself a people for his own possession who are zealous for good works." Knowing that man is a sinner, God provided a way that he could be redeemed, and live above the lawless state he had originally thrust himself into. However, it is important for man to accept God's free gift, or there will be no assurance of the same. Please consider Romans 10:10: "For with the heart one believes and is justified, and with the mouth one confesses and is saved."

One of the reasons for providing redemption through the work of Jesus is that ordinary people— like you and me—may be brought back into a proper relationship with God. God, our Maker, designed people with both physical and spiritual dimensions. Jesus Himself, born of Mary, came into the world in a physical body. He ate food, drank liquids, grew physically, and attained various stages of physical, social and spiritual maturity. Luke 2:52 records that "Jesus increased in wisdom and in stature and in favor with God and man."

Soul and Body—Both Are Important

The Bible unashamedly presents people as having both physical and spiritual aspects in their design. Both the Old Testament and the New Testament look forward to a final state in which we will live in perfect, resurrected bodies.

Even though we presently live in a world in which decay and death are ever-present realities, the Bible encourages a healthy and positive view of our physical makeup. Jesus took great care to heal and restore people as He went about doing good. He commissioned His apostles to do some of the same kinds of things. And after the times transitioned from His three-year ministry to the crucifixion and resurrection, the body of Jesus did not lie for long in the grave. In His real human body He ascended to heaven, and He will one day come back in that same, resurrected, glorified body!

The great preacher and Christian medical doctor, D. Martyn Lloyd-Jones, made the point that it is a less-than-Christian view that considers matter—and especially the human body—as evil or unworthy of proper care and attention.[1] In the times after the New Testament was written, there were some wrong views in circulation in which people believed that spirit was essentially good, and that matter—physical stuff, including the body—was essentially evil. This led to some wrong thinking about the human body, sometimes being worked out in gluttony, sexual immorality, or at times in an ascetic lifestyle in which bodily needs and cares were largely ignored or played down.

At another extreme, too much emphasis was placed on the body strong and beautiful. Some thinking and teaching that the Greeks embraced made the physical self a kind of idol to be held in awe and reverence.

The Bible's Balanced View

The Bible is superbly balanced in the way it considers the interplay between the spiritual and the physical. God is Spirit, and there is a significant spiritual realm; nevertheless, He has made humans as psychosomatic beings—which means that their makeup includes spiritual and material aspects—and both require attention in living in a way that is pleasing to Him. Consequently, it is important to care for one's body and so be continually fit for His use.

This sets the scene for us to consider the emphasis of the key references from the Old and New Testaments.

- 1 Corinthians 16: 19-20 states: "... Do you not know that your body is a temple of the Holy Spirit within you, whom you have from God? You are not your own, for you were bought with a price. So glorify God in your body."

- 1 Timothy 4:8 records: "For while bodily training is of some value, godliness is of value in every way, as it holds promise for the present life and also for the life to come."

- Ephesians 5:18 says, "And do not get drunk with wine, for that is debauchery, but be filled with the Spirit." We should be responsible with our bodies, especially being careful with what we put in them, and considering the outcomes that could result.

- 1 Corinthians 15:54-58 states: "When the perishable puts on the imperishable, and the mortal puts on immortality, then shall come to pass the saying that is written: 'Death is swallowed up in victory.' 'O death, where is your victory? O death, where is your sting?' The sting of death is sin, and the power of sin is the law. But thanks be to God, who gives us the victory through our Lord Jesus Christ. Therefore, my beloved brothers, be steadfast, immovable, always abounding in the work of the Lord, knowing that in the Lord your labor is not in vain." Read the whole of 1 Corinthians 15 and its teaching on the resurrection of our bodies to see how important, from God's perspective, our bodies actually are!

- Jeremiah 9:23-24 states "Thus says the LORD: 'Let not the wise man boast in his wisdom, let not the mighty man boast in his might, let not the rich man boast in his riches, but let him who boasts boast in this, that he understands and knows me, that I am the LORD who practices steadfast love, justice, and righteousness in the earth. For in these things I delight, declares the LORD.'"

- Psalm 18:30-34 says, "This God—his way is perfect; the word of the LORD proves true;   he is a shield for all those who take refuge in him. For who is God, but the LORD? And who is a rock, except our God?—the God who equipped me with strength and made my way blameless. He made my feet like the feet of a deer and set me secure on the heights. He trains my hands for war, so that my arms can bend a bow of bronze."

- Psalm 144:1 says, "Blessed be the LORD, my rock, who trains my hands for war, and my fingers for battle."

- 1 Peter 5:5 states that we are to "clothe ourselves in humility." In all of one's consideration for weights and conditioning, it is still important to recognize what Galatians 6:14 says: "But far be it from me to boast except in the cross of our Lord Jesus Christ, by which the world has been crucified to me, and I to the world."

- 2 Corinthians 10:12 says that "when they measure themselves by one another and compare themselves with one another, they are without understanding." Galatians 6:3 makes the point that "if anyone thinks he is something, when he is nothing, he deceives himself."

Putting All of This Together...

For Christians, it is important to note that their bodies are considered to be temples of the Holy Spirit (1 Corinthians 6:19). In the Bible, the temple was understood to be a place where God was especially present. The connection in thought is vitally important: if you are a believer—if your faith and trust are in Christ to be your Savior and you are endeavoring to live a life pleasing to Him—then your body is a dwelling place for the Holy Spirit! If you care for your own residence (whether a family home, apartment or condo)—and surely you do, taking the time and trouble to maintain it, remodel it from time to time, decorating it when it needs such attention— then how much more should you take care of the physical body God has entrusted to you!

To extend this analogy, of course moderation is a key consideration. The Bible calls for moderation in all things ("Let your moderation be known unto all men"—see Philippians 4:5, KJV). There is a time and a place for everything (Ecclesiastes 3:1–8). The careful and controlled pursuit of bodily exercise, in endeavoring to be fit for the Master, doing all things heartily as to Him (Colossians 3:23) may be a vital component in your usefulness to Him as you live out the days and years He has appointed for you in this world.

The Christian Perspective
Living in our modern society can be challenging, especially as there is such a culture of competition to be thin and/or muscular and/or beautiful (etc.) in order to feel a significant sense of self-worth. People focusing on such externals will not find their fulfillment in Jesus and His purposes. The message of Jesus is so different: He is the source of self-worth;

you don't need to find it in superficial and socially related things. Your relationship with Him, not the way you look or how much you weigh, should mean the most to you as a Christian.

Yes, it can be hard to live outside of society's standards! Yet, Christ never gave in to that pressure. He lived in the world, but He was not of the world. The aim of a Christian is to be like Christ. The ultimate message He sends is that He loves His people unconditionally, and He therefore wants you to consider yourself in the light of that. As one person said, "God doesn't make any junk."

In reading the final part of this chapter, consider the following biblical principles and references:

- The Lord Jesus Christ, in coming into this world, did so not as an angel or some kind of spirit, but as the God-Man. Philippians 2 and 1 Timothy 3:16 make it clear that the Second Person of the Trinity became fully human and, in His body, achieved redemption for ordinary people. God's grace to us was brought through the physical, bodily suffering, death and resurrection of Jesus. Soldiers slammed nails through his hands and feet, ripping through skin, tendons, and muscle. They smashed a crown of thorns on his head. They stabbed a spear into his side, and bodily fluids poured out. Jesus died on a rugged cross. He went through it, suffering in his body because people are made up of both body and soul. Jesus had to really die, to provide a blood sacrifice, so that people, after seeking forgiveness for their sins, might have eternal life. To accomplish this redemption, Jesus had to be both fully man and fully God.

- People are wonderfully created in God's image, after His likeness. While this may be primarily a spiritual reference, the fact is that He has placed us in bodies. These bodies are to be offered up to Him in the process of living a life of practical usefulness in this world. Romans 12:1 urges us: "I appeal to you therefore, brothers, by the mercies of God, to present your bodies as a living sacrifice, holy and acceptable to God, which is your spiritual worship."

- A healthy body is one that enables you more easily and practically to glorify God.

- Adam and Eve, and all of their descendents, were created in the image of God, to be busy working in and stewards over creation. Caring for one's physical body is one of these creative tasks.

- Modern society's view of beauty is one that is very different from the one the Bible emphasizes. As God's image bearers, in whatever way He has made our physical form, we do have a beauty, and our sense of self-worth is tied in with this. Never believe the lie that says you are ugly!

- John 10:10 makes the point that Jesus came so that we may have life, and have it to the full. John later wished his readers good health in writing these words: "Beloved, I pray that all may go well with you and that you may be in good health, as it goes well with your soul" (3 John 2).

You are fearfully and wonderfully made in the image of God, the Master Creator. You can achieve a measure of health and fitness, and enjoy the purpose for which you have been made. Read on to find out more!

2

Health and a Healthy Self-Image

Enjoying being the "you" that God intends you to be

O LORD, you have searched me and known me!
You know when I sit down and when I rise up;
you discern my thoughts from afar. You search out my
path and my lying down
and are acquainted with all my ways.
Even before a word is on my tongue,
behold, O LORD, you know it altogether.

(Psalm 139:1–4)

Created Strong

God has created man with the ability to exercise. There are many references to physical activity in the Bible and to sports in the New Testament. Through the apostle Paul, God addresses the matter as a question "Do you not know that in a race all the runners run, but only one receives the prize?" (1 Corinthians 9:24a). However, He also says, "So run that you may obtain it." (1 Corinthians 9:24b). Elsewhere, using a physical analogy, He says that no man having put his hand to the plow and looking back is fit for the kingdom of heaven (Luke 9:62). That context has to do with farming and the physical exertion that is undertaken when one is plowing a field. In another passage, Paul says, "I press on toward the goal for the prize of the upward call of God in Christ Jesus" (Philippians 3:14).

From an historical point of view, sports such as the Olympic Games provide an excellent resource for illustrations. People would exert themselves and compete for a wreath that faded quickly away (1 Corinthians 9:25). In no way is exercise or fitness to be something that is lauded merely for its own sake. We exercise and physically exert ourselves for a purpose; in the Olympic Games, candidates ran to win. Intentionality was called for.

Since believers are described as being temples of the Holy Spirit—places where He personally resides—it is important that these temples become physically fit for His use. It is a biblical principle that faithfulness is rewarded. Everyone who pursues faithfulness can attain it.

Ruined by the Fall

Most people grow and mature to full strength by about the time they are twenty-five years old. It is documented that peak physical condition is achieved at this stage.[2] If life consists, as Scripture calls it, of three score and ten years—that is, seventy years (see Psalm 90)—that means that the body from age twenty-five on does not continue to improve but actually begins to deteriorate. As in anything, when something is left to itself, it will begin the process of atrophy. That is not to say that a person who is committed to keeping fit is guaranteed a long and healthy life, but it does mean that not exercising is beginning a process where the body is no longer as fit for God's use as it would be if exercise were routinely undertaken.

Fitness Can Help

What does fitness produce? One major ingredient that only comes about through exercise—and is produced directly within our bodies—is that of endorphins. Endorphins are energy-released chemicals that enhance our physical makeup as well as contribute greatly to our general approach to life.

God consistently says that we are to rejoice always and be thankful (1 Thessalonians 5:16, 18). It is possible to mentally will that to occur, and many times that is necessary. However, if one can enhance that will with a body that is fit—one in which endorphins are being released—it makes it so much easier to actually have that positive outlook.

Through medical research, people have developed drugs that can stimulate muscle growth or strength. Often these are considered illegal because such may be enhancing drugs—substances that make people go beyond their regular physical limitations to become stronger or faster. However, after consecutive doses of such a manmade drug and its use is stopped, the body becomes debilitated and will be worse off than before. Because such substances can be addictive, the user may find that he has to continue using them on a consistent basis, otherwise he is not going to feel well. Many people take drugs to make them go to sleep; others take drugs to help them wake up in the morning. In many cases, by implementing exercise into their daily routines, such people can manage without those types of drugs.

God has said that man will toil and by the sweat of his brow he will work (see Genesis 3:17–19). That physical toil brings him to exhaustion. A measure of exhaustion causes a person to enjoy a good night's sleep. And a good, proper night's sleep will bring one to a state of refreshment. Drug-induced sleep does not produce the same quality of rest as physically exhausted daily living will. And the same goes for taking medications to improve alertness during the day—it is far better to have rested well during the night than to depend on a substance in order to be efficient during daylight hours!

Not only does sleep come so much more easily to a person who has exerted his body, but it is interesting to know that a person in a fit state needs not quite as much sleep. Just like a well-maintained engine in a vehicle operates so much more smoothly and uses less gas for the work it does, a body that is generally in a fit state will not need as much refreshment to be charged and ready to function the next day. You can read more about this in Chapter 7.

It is interesting to note that the industry of drugs and medicines and stimulants is becoming more and more prevalent as our society becomes more and more sedentary. It is often so that people would rather eat or somehow ingest their rest by mouth than to take the rest that God actually provides through sleep. People enjoy staying up for entertainment purposes but then find it difficult getting proper rest because their bodies are not fit and exhausted. They feel they need something to get them charged up for the next day to be able to function properly. Our world has so many energy drinks and energy enhancements available and those who use them—even if they contain toxins—find that these products initially have a positive effect on them. However, in reality, the chemicals found in these products are not going to naturally help these individuals be what they could be.

So if energy drinks and stimulants are not really helpful, what is the answer? The natural and God-given way is exercise and rest. Both of these should be in proper proportion and in moderation. It is wrong to say that a little exercise is good so lots of exercise makes it even better. Rather, one should find what helps make one's body the most efficient for God's glory. Taking into consideration the natural cycle of a day, it is evident that from the beginning, when God created the sun, moon and stars, He established the pattern of mornings and evenings, days and nights. He knew that when He created human beings, they were going to need to function on a daily cycle. That cycle has unfortunately been stretched and distorted today because of the conveniences of electricity, and a result of the means by which people can use electronic media and be stimulated for a lot longer than is good for them.

If people would realize their goal in life is to love God and bring glory to Him, then they would take that as their lifelong approach and desire to do so all the day long. Therefore, when it relates to fitness, it requires them to evaluate their entire life and to determine what is going to help them best to be able to function for God's glory.

Joy, Endorphins and the Manufacturer's Handbook

God has created our bodies in such a way that they are able to withstand pressure and be strengthened when pressure is applied. That pressure comes in a variety of ways. One way (the way this book will direct you) is that of exercise. Exercise will strengthen the heart. The heart, by being strengthened, will beat fewer beats per minute and will function more efficiently. By beating fewer times and more efficiently, it is going to be able to beat longer. That allows for one's physical makeup from the blood flow to be in better condition and for one to be able to live more efficiently for God's use.

Medical specialists have determined certain blood pressure values that identify whether one is in an overall state of good health—in the region of 120/70. They have also determined how many heart beats a minute is the standard for people typically in good health—between 60 and 80 beats per minute. God's Word, the Bible, encourages individuals to cultivate lifestyles that are conducive to their wellbeing, so it is helpful to consider the reference points supplied by medical specialists and be guided by such parameters. Whether a person is a student, an employee, a homemaker or retired—whatever a person's calling may be—it is important to be in as good a state of health and with as high a level of energy as possible.

The Bible often addresses life by way of broad principles, so there are no Scripture references that speak specifically to bed times and participating in exercise. However, scientists and other medical specialists have found that increased exercise and regulated sleep have the effect of enhancing many of the things that people do. Science—and keep in mind that true science is simply accurate knowledge—confirms the wisdom of building good habits in these areas.

God created humans as physical beings, and declared everything that He had created was good. In caring for the garden, Adam was to be involved in physical work. When endorphins are released in response to physical activity, there is a direct correlation on the part of the person exercising in that he or she has a much more thrilling and enjoyable experience of life. While the Bible nowhere explains how or why endorphins are released in response to physical exertion, the fact of the matter is this: people engaging in physical activity typically enjoy heightened euphoric feelings, and therefore a significant sense of wellbeing. Exercise (keep in mind that exercise involves exertion) releases these endorphins. So, people who pursue endorphin-releasing activities have this sense of joy and peace.

People will often comment on the joy, laughter, and energy that children have. Have you ever heard a statement like, "I would like to bottle some of that energy and have it for myself"? Children are known to enjoy playing. They don't look at the clock and determine they have too much to do so they cannot play. They simply play and enjoy life. That play undoubtedly involves exertion, which in turn triggers the release of endorphins.

As children grow into teenagers and adults, unfortunately play is not something that they are able to do as often. Life begins to form into larger work segments. Even school is work. That is one reason why physical activity in a school is so important. Whether it's inter-school competition or intra-school competition, it is good for there to be a means of outlet for the students through physical exertion. That exertion is what brings the opportunity to have this sense of wellbeing and a better joyful outlook on their life.

As people's activity levels diminish, they may still willfully and intentionally be joyful people, but even that can wear off. Being joyful does not make one fit. Being fit, however, will easily translate into having a joy-filled life. Therefore, it is extremely important to consider how to be joy filled amidst the pressures of life.

The control of exercise, though, must be considered as well. Our modern society allows for way too much emphasis on the body. People, God's image-bearers, may be tempted to place a disproportionate emphasis on their bodies, flaunting and perverting them. The 1980 movie, *Fame*, captured something of this in the song "I sing the body electric":

> I sing the body electric,
> I celebrate the me yet to come;
> I toast to my own reunion,
> When I become one with the sun!

It is a vitally important principle: God wants us to be godly with contentment—the Bible's position is that bodily training has value (see 1 Timothy 4:8). Exercise enhances the body, so if that body is to be used for God's glory—which was His intention from the beginning—then the focus of the exercise is to help us be more fit for God's use. To desire to have a fit body just for its own sake (not considering our responsibility and duty to serve God) is to put the cart before the horse. Bodily exercise is profitable, for it does bring one into a state of greater fitness, but it is not merely fitness in itself that is going to ultimately bring God glory. God is glorified when we find contentment in whatever state He has placed us. This involves our loving Him first and foremost and loving others also—see Matthew 22:38.

Making It Happen...

Another great benefit that exercise provides is in positioning people in the community, where they can be salt and light in the world. While Christians should realize that their fitness is for God's glory, they are able to be with those whose goal in fitness is for their own benefit only. Here, believers may make a strong impact on unconverted friends and associates as they demonstrate how it is possible in the first place to love and serve the living God, and yet also desire to be fit and healthy. Their lives are a testimony to the truth of the Word of God as they live it out in day-to-day life. God wants people to love Him and desire Him because He is worthy of that, not because He's going to do anything for them!

Because God has not created all people in the same way, there will be a range of exercises that will help people in different ways. It is therefore important to assess one's strengths and weaknesses, and to consider what would be most appropriate in achieving greater fitness.

God wants people to do all things in moderation. There is a time and a season for everything, so exercise is not to outweigh work. Neither should work outweigh time with family. And time with family is not to outweigh rest. It can be challenging to work out the details of how to do things in moderation. But if God says that we can do all things through Him as He strengthens us, then we can do all things to bring glory to Him.

In this respect, it is important to be sure that you are taking the long-term view and defining your goals in life. Once you have determined that you want to bring God glory, you need to find what will most enhance your life so you may best do that. If you find goals that you really desire but also that there are obstacles that will keep you from those goals, be sure to assess whether your goals are too high or the obstacles are too frightening. There is a way that you can follow that will bring God glory, and He will enable you as you seek Him and His strength to do so!

Get Medical Clearance
One last point: it will always be extremely important to have medical clearance prior to engaging in a

significant physical activity. Qualified and licensed medical personnel are well able to assess the needs and capabilities of individuals. Be sure to pay attention to such recommendations!

3

You Don't Have to Over-Strain!

Understanding the place of exercise

For you formed my inward parts;
you knitted me together in my mother's womb.
I praise you, for I am fearfully and wonderfully made.
Wonderful are your works;
my soul knows it very well.
My frame was not hidden from you,
when I was being made in secret,
intricately woven in the depths of the earth.
Your eyes saw my unformed substance;
in your book were written, every one of them,
the days that were formed for me,
when as yet there was none of them.

(Psalm 139:13–16)

A Case Study

Researchers Peter Walters and John Byl have reported elevated mood and reduced anxiety and depression in candidates after exercise. The main reason for this is the release of chemical substances by the body during exercise. These endorphins act as opiates, and they decrease pain as well as produce feelings of wellbeing.

Research undertaken by Walters and Byl suggests that exercise can be effective treatment for clinical depression. A study was done on twenty-four patients diagnosed with moderate depression. This group was subdivided into either an exercise group or psychotherapy group. The group that received psychotherapy met with a psychologist once a week, while the exercise group went jogging with a trainer three times a week for 45 to 60 minutes.

After twelve weeks, about three fourths of the patients in each of the groups had recovered from their depression. That means that in both categories they had recovered. However, after one year, half of those in the psychotherapy group returned for additional depression treatment, while none of the subjects in the exercise group returned.

Exercising Naturally

Exercise is something most people can incorporate naturally into their daily or weekly schedules. When considering getting into good physical shape—and staying there—it will be important to establish certain guidelines to always try to meet. By doing so, it will become a part of your life rather than a drudgery or something that has to be checked off a to-do list.

As researcher Laura Larsen has confirmed, exercise has life-changing benefits.[3] Very often, people like to repeat the famous quotation "No pain, no gain!" which is really a way of stating an old-fashioned way of thinking. Yet, current health studies prove that exercise doesn't have to hurt to be incredibly effective. Research indicates that even short intervals of exercise may be a powerful tool to super-charge your health. By making it a way of life, you will enjoy so much more exercise in a natural way, and it is likely that it won't even involve your putting it into segments. Some benefits of exercise are the following.

The Benefits of Exercise[4]

- Exercise relieves stress and anxiety.

- Exercise alleviates depression. Exercise treats mild to moderate depression as effectively as antidepressant medicines. Experts believe that physical activity releases serotonin, a brain chemical that fights negative thoughts and depression.

- Exercise improves our mood. As has been mentioned, exercise also releases endorphins, powerful chemicals in our brain that energize our spirits and simply make us feel good.

- Exercise sharpens our brainpower. The same endorphins that make us feel better also help us concentrate and feel mentally sharp for a task that may be at hand.

- Exercise improves our self-esteem. Regular activity is an investment in your mind, body, and soul. When it becomes a habit, it can help foster a stronger sense of self-worth since you take the time to take care of yourself.

- Exercise assists in energy gain. It is amazing that, no matter how often you may feel tired or may not desire to exercise, the exercise actually has the effect of rejuvenating you!

Myths about Exercise

Exercise also has some myths associated with it. Consider the following list:

- "Working out once a week won't help." The fact is some exercise is always better than none. The small amount of exercise can often help you maintain or get into more of an active routine. Try to continue the low or mediocre amount of exercise you are accustomed to doing until you can gradually add more dates.

- "No pain, no gain." Have you ever heard it said that if working out doesn't hurt it isn't working? The fact is strenuous exercise may make you breathe heavily and your muscles may ache temporarily, but exercise should not be painful. In fact, if it is, it may indicate an injury or muscle strain. Many forms of exercise, like walking, swimming, or gentle stretching, get results without discomfort.

- "Exercise tires you out." People often already feel exhausted and believe that working out will just make it worse. The fact is that physical activity actually makes you more alert. The endorphins that are released relax your body and energize your mind.

- "Exercise is not going to stop a person from getting older, so why bother?" While exercise cannot turn back the clock, it can make your body healthier and stronger. People who exercise regularly feel better and can move as if they were younger.

Types of Cardiorespiratory Exercise

The type of exercise is important in an individual's process of becoming fit. Exercise is so important because of how it intersects and interfaces between body and soul. In particular, if the heart is well exercised, it is usually a straightforward matter to keep the rest of the body well regulated.

Various exercises are characterized by different levels of impact involved. As a general principle, for a person in reasonable health, high-impact exercises are efficient in building bone and muscle strength, as well as overall body toning. High-impact exercises are generally more vigorous, and because of this, effort is efficiently expended. Results appear relatively quickly. Many people find brisk walking an easy way to start and become acclimated to the exercise process.

In achieving the best outcomes from exercise,

there are four considerations to keep in mind: Frequency, intensity, time and type.[5] These four elements are interconnected. A person starting an exercise program through a series of routine walks will find that as his or her aerobic capacity increases, so will the ability to work longer, more frequently, and with greater intensity. This is seen in the following scenario:

- Frequency: He aims to exercise five times per week;
- Intensity: in the long term, he might aim to double his heart rate on each of these occasions—see the paragraph below these bullet points.
- Time: He is sure to work himself for time periods of twenty minutes;
- Type: He selects a type of activity that incorporates different muscle groups for a sustained period of time.

Initially, begin your exercise program so you that gradually increase your heart rate. This may take six months or more if you are just a beginner. Eventually a fit person may double his or her heartbeat and be able to hold it at that level for at least twenty minutes, three times a week. Cardiorespiratory exercise has the capacity to raise heart rate to a level at which an aerobic benefit can occur. The following section describes some of the more popular forms of aerobic exercises. Don't limit your cardio options to these activities, though. There are many forms of cardiorespiratory exercise, and the most important aspect is to find one that you will enjoy and that will have the proper frequency, intensity, and time to yield benefits in your life.

- *Walking* is a low-impact activity that may be the most convenient form of activity in existence. Walkers can exercise almost any time, in any type of weather condition, with practically no special exercise equipment.

- *Jogging* is an exercise that numerous people say they participate in. Jogging can also be done at almost any time and any type of weather but is considered a high-impact activity as opposed to low-impact activity.

- *Swimming*, a no-impact activity, is another very important consideration for cardiorespiratory exercise. Of course to swim, one must have learned at least the American crawl stroke! Breaststroke and backstroke are good to use, too. By using those large muscle groups and propelling oneself in the water, much intensity can occur with very low impact.

- *Cycling* is an exercise which, of course, must be done on a bicycle. Again, this exercise can be done in most weather conditions but there is always the consideration of where to cycle. From an efficiency point of view, it also takes about three times the number of exercise minutes to reap the same benefit as running would yield.
- *Other* very valuable aerobic exercises can be achieved by using cardiorespiratory equipment. This includes elliptical machines, Stairmasters, stationary bikes, rowing machines, and any other types of equipment that get a person's heart rate to the level necessary for aerobic conditioning.

The Heart of the Matter

Your heart ensures that essential oxygen and nutrients are transported to the various parts of your body. As a general rule, the better your heart works, the better shape you are in. The good news is that it is possible to keep your heart healthy by engaging routinely in exercise. There are several very distinct advantages to having cardiorespiratory exercise.

- The *first* is it fights heart disease. In a study (conducted by Larsen) of over 2,500 adult men, those who walked for just thirty minutes a day reduced their risk of heart disease by almost 50 percent.

- *Second*, cholesterol can also be reduced through cardiorespiratory exercise. Many studies have been done on how eating oat bran can lower blood cholesterol. One study demonstrated that if a person consistently followed that diet, a 1 percent drop in cholesterol would be the outcome. Compare that, however, to the average cardiovascular exercise, which is much more effective and is able to lower blood cholesterol by as much as 24 percent.

- A *third* result of cardiorespiratory exercise—because it promotes health—is that it enhances the body's immune function. This is a result of increasing the body's ability to fight off diseases simply because it is more fit and capable.

Setting Goals

Once you have made the decision to become more aerobically fit, it is very important to set a goal and have this accomplished. Proverbs 13:12 speaks how unfulfilled expectations can bring discouragement. However, verse 19 says "the desire fulfilled is sweet to the soul." It is possible to become discouraged at any time. Most often, people become discouraged are when their goals have not been fulfilled. Some of those have been goals that they have set out to accomplish, whereas others have been those they broadly hoped would happen. Nonetheless "hope deferred makes the heart sick." To have a desire fulfilled, it is important to outline an aerobic exercise plan and this must include the following:

Set an overall goal. That goal may be to run, cycle, swim (or whatever exercise may have been determined), and to do it for a certain distance. Once that has been determined, then you next need to determine how many times a week to participate in that activity. It is best to set, as a minimum threshold, exercising three times a week for twenty minutes.

Establish the right level of intensity. Intensity is another aspect to be considered when exercising. Intensity may be one of the most important factors in developing your cardiorespiratory fitness. It is easy to make mistakes in one of two ways: if you don't push yourself hard enough, you won't improve; on the other hand, if you push yourself too hard, you'll be susceptible to exercise-related injuries.

Do the math carefully. There are several ways to determine an appropriate zone for aerobic exercise. The two that will be discussed here involve (a) determining your estimated maximum heart rate and then pursuing a certain rate for exertion or (b) to actually use a heart rate monitor which allows you to review your progress in real time as you exert yourself.

Follow these steps to calculate the best way to exercise your heart.

- The first calculation of your heart rate involves calculating your estimated maximum heart rate. You do this by subtracting your age from 220. If you're 31 years old, for example, your estimated maximum heart rate would be 189 beats per minute (bpm). You can tell from this formula that your maximum heart rate decreases with age.
- Next you determine the lower and upper limit that falls within a range of percentage of your estimated maximum heart rate. The aim is to work hard enough to maintain or increase cardiorespiratory function without working to the point of injury or dread of exercise because it is so painful.
- Understand that exercising at less than 40 percent

of maximum heart rate won't provide sufficient cardiorespiratory stress to increase or maintain fitness and health. The American College of Sports Medicine established 55 to 65 percent of maximum heart rate as the minimum intensity level for aerobic exercise. For those who are apparently healthy, 65 to 90 percent is recommended. This means that 65 percent of your maximum heart rate should be the minimum that is achieved during exercise and that 90 percent of the maximum heart rate would be the maximum.

- An example for the 31-year-old shows that the estimated maximum heart rate is 189. The lower limit is 123 bpm which is determined by multiplying 189×65 percent. The upper limit is 170 bpm which is achieved by multiplying 189×90 percent.

The second calculation for the training heart rate zone is to use a heart rate monitor. By knowing the formula for achieving a heart rate, one is able to determine the minimum or maximum by observing the heart rate monitor as it displays the exact numeric value. The heart rate monitor requires you to have a chest strap with a sensor that measures your heart's beating rate per minute and that reveals the number on a portable display unit such as a watch face.

Practical Tips for Getting Started in an Exercise Program

It's easier to work out when you have started to be in good shape. And the good news is that, even if you're starting at Ground Zero, you can still work out! Exercise is the only way to help you get in shape. If you have no exercise experience, you can start slowly with low-impact movements a few minutes each day and then continue to improve and increase these.

- *Take it slowly.* The best thing you can do to ease yourself into a fitness plan is to take a moderate and carefully thought through approach. Trying to achieve too much too soon may lead to frustrations and injuries. So, start with what you feel comfortable with. For example, training for a marathon when you've never run before may be a bit daunting, but you could set yourself the goal of participating in an upcoming 5-kilometer walk or run.

- *Schedule your exercise.* People don't go to important meetings and appointments spontaneously; rather, they schedule them. If you have trouble fitting exercise into your schedule, consider it an important appointment with yourself, and mark it on your daily or weekly agenda.

- *Be realistic and expect ups and downs.* Don't be discouraged if you skip a few days or even a few weeks while you get the process underway. These interruptions will happen. Just get started again and slowly build up your momentum

Safety Tips for When You Begin to Exercise

It's important to go into an exercise program carefully and thoughtfully. Key safety tips for you to keep in mind as you begin to exercise are as follows.

- *Make sure you have medical clearance.* Your physician should be able to guide you in this matter, especially if you do have background health concerns. Many insurance companies offer free checkups, so do take care in this regard, and only pursue an exercise program if you are given proper medical clearance.

- *Be sure you stretch.* Do your stretches incrementally to avoid trauma. You can do this by starting with gentle stretching, and then gradually extend the pattern.

- *Keep drinking plenty of water.* Be sure to be

hydrated before you start. If you are thirsty when you start, you are already dehydrated. Exercise can make you sweat, so you need to take extra care not to dehydrate!

Make the Time; Take the Time!

Time is a factor in exercising. It really doesn't take a big investment in time to improve aerobic fitness, especially when beginning an exercise program. One study showed that aerobic fitness improved in low-fitness subjects with as little as ten minutes of cardiorespiratory exercise per day. In another study, only five minutes of daily, high-intensity exercise caused an increase in cardiorespiratory performance. Although very short bouts of exercise are beneficial to someone just starting out, longer sessions are better for those with some experience. The American College of Sports Medicine recommends 20 to 60 minutes of aerobic exercise per session, excluding warm-up and cool-down time.

Thomas Jefferson once said, "You can make time for exercise now, or you can make time for sickness later!"

4

Exercise Guidelines

Developing a practical strategy that suits you

Rather train yourself for godliness; for while bodily training is of some value, godliness is of value in every way, as it holds promise for the present life and also for the life to come.

(1 Timothy 4:7–8)

I n many studies covering a wide range of issues, researchers have focused on exercise as well as on the more broadly defined concept of physical activity. Exercise is a form of physical activity as planned, structured, repetitive, and performed with the goal of improving health or fitness. So although all exercise is physical activity, not all physical activity is exercise.

This book is intended to encourage everyone to be fit for the Master's use. God created us, and therefore we should be as functional as possible, so bringing Him glory while being able to lead more efficient and effective lives.

Three Divisions in Exercise

When one considers physical fitness, it is important to keep in mind three types of exercising and the specific applications associated with them. They are aerobic activity, muscle strengthening activity, and bone strengthening activity.

Aerobic Activity is the kind of physical activity which helps the body's large muscles move in a rhythmic manner for a sustained period of time. Brisk walking, running, bicycling, using a jumping rope, and swimming are all examples of aerobic activity that cause a person's heart to beat faster than usual. This simply strengthens the heart so that, as an outcome, it does not need to beat as often as that of a sedentary person. This, in turn, enhances such a person's fitness level.

Aerobic activity has three components, as follows.
- *Frequency*, or how often a person does aerobic activity.
- *Intensity*, or how hard a person works to do the activity.
- *Time*, or how long a person does an activity in any one session.
- *Type*, or the specific activity chosen for exercise.[6]

Although these components make up a physical activity profile, research has shown that the total measure of physical activity is more important in achieving health benefits than is any single component (that is, frequency, intensity, or time). The bottom line to successful aerobic activity is simply doing it!

Muscle Strengthening Activity: A second kind of physical activity is *muscle strengthening activity*. This kind of activity includes resistance training and lifting weights, and causes the body's muscles to work or hold something against an applied force or weight. These activities often use relatively heavy objects, such as weights, which are lifted multiple times to train and strengthen various muscle groups. Muscle strengthening, however, can also be done by using elastic bands or body weight for resistance. Even doing yard work is valuable.

Muscle strengthening activity also has three components.

- *Intensity*, or how much weight or force is used relative to how much a person is able to exert.
- *Frequency*, or how often a person does muscle strengthening activity
- *Repetitions*, or how many times a person lifts a weight.

The effects of muscle strengthening activity are limited to muscles doing the work. Therefore, it is important to work all the major muscle groups of the body—the legs, hips, back, abdomen, chest, shoulders, and arms.

Bone Strengthening Activity: Finally it is important for there to be a *bone strengthening activity*. This kind of activity (sometimes called weight-bearing or weight loading activity) produces a force in the bones that promotes bone growth and strength. This force is commonly produced by impact with the ground. Examples of bone strengthening activity include jumping jacks, running, brisk walking, and weight lifting exercises. As these examples illustrate, bone strengthening activities can also be aerobic and muscle strengthening in nature.

Since there is a principle that all things should be done in moderation, it is important to consider bodily exercise and to follow the practice of improving one's cardiovascular condition. By doing so, one can be even more fit for the Master's use. Exercise, all in all, will improve a person's physical condition thus enabling him or her to live more efficiently, and allowing one's physical makeup to operate more effectively.

Optimizing Your Physical Activity
The beneficial effects of increasing physical activity

are threefold: it's about *overload, progression*, and *specificity*.

Overload is the physical stress placed on the body where physical activity is greater in its measure of intensity than usual. The body structures and functions respond and adapt to these stresses. For example, aerobic physical activity places a stress on the cardiorespiratory system and muscles, requiring the lungs to move air, and the heart to pump more blood and deliver it to the working muscles. This increase in demand enlarges the efficiency and capacity of the lungs, heart, circulatory system, and exercising muscles. In the same way, muscle strengthening and bone strengthening activities overload muscles and bones, making them stronger.

Progression is closely tied to overload. Once a person reaches a certain physical fitness level, he or she progresses to higher levels of physical activity by continued overload and adaptation. Small, progressive changes in overload help the body adapt to the additional stresses, therefore minimizing the risk of injury.

Specificity means that the benefits of physical exercise are specific to the body systems that are doing the work. For example, aerobic physical activity largely benefits the body's cardiovascular system. People gain health and fitness by being habitually physically active. The benefits of physical activity also outweigh the risk of injury and sudden heart attacks, two concerns that many people are worried about when it comes to physical activity.

Research by Penny Stanway has established a link between moderate, regular exercise on the one hand, and a strong immune system on the other.[7] Early studies showed that people engaging in recreational exercises reported succumbing to fewer colds once they had begun the practice of jogging. Moderate exercise has been linked to a positive immune system response and the temporary boost in cells that attack bacteria. It is believed that regular, consistent exercise can lead to substantial benefits and immune system health over the long term.

However, just as important as exercise is, there is evidence that too much intense exercise can reduce a person's immunity. That is one reason why it is so important to do this in moderation.

A practical word of counsel is worth highlighting here: Everyone is going to get sick at some time. So, the question is, should one then still exercise? The rule of thumb is that if the illness is not related to a fever, then moderate exercise will still have its benefits. However, exercising with a fever can be physically harmful and should not be done.

How Much Should I Exercise, and What Exercise Is Best?

Once a person realizes the purpose and importance of exercise and implements a course of action, the next question to answer is this: How much is enough?

A biblical principle with a practical outworking is that we are to do all things in a balanced way. This means that, on the one hand, we need some exercise so that we are at least doing it in moderation, but, on the other hand, we are not becoming excessive. Most people do not move or exercise sufficiently for it to be of benefit. But what is "enough"? This may vary from person to person. First of all, consider the need for health, fitness, and athletic performance and determine clearly what it is that should be achieved. Then, decide how much is needed and realistically implement a plan to reach such goals. Many people simply wish to achieve a measure of good health.

Health may seem to be the most achievable goal, but in reality health is quite a difficult term to define. Perhaps the best way to understand it is actually by its absence. If chosen wisely, a range of activities can improve your health.

While exercise can improve health, fitness is something else. Health and fitness, however, are often automatically associated with each other. If you ask an exercise physiologist, you will be told that fitness refers to cardiovascular or cardiorespiratory fitness or aerobic capacity. Physical fitness, in this sense, is a measure of how efficiently you transport oxygen to laboring muscles and maintain movement. A physically fit person has strong lungs, a robust heart, and sturdy muscles. However, that person may or may not be clinically healthy. Some people blessed with high marks in fitness can have miserable cholesterol profiles or even rotund waistlines!

A surprisingly large measure of any person's biological fitness is, in fact, innate. According to several large recent studies, 30 percent or more of a person's cardiovascular fitness may be genetic. You are born either more or less physically fit than the next person. But, how you enhance or diminish that inheritance is up to you.

Being sure to exercise in bite-sizes each day is one way of getting there. Even just committing to three sessions of ten minutes at a time each day can have an excellent cumulative value. Walking three miles a day on a regular basis will almost certainly improve most your health and fitness. Running four marathons in a year might not.

What this means, in laymen's terms, is that, according to the best available science, you should walk, or otherwise work out, for 150 minutes a week in order to improve your health. This report (undertaken by Laura Larsen) shows that you can split those 150 minutes into almost any number of chunks and still benefit. In a study of aerospace engineers, who were first-time exercisers, the men were assigned to briskly walk or urgently jog for 30 minutes a day in either a single, uninterrupted half hour, or in three 10-minute sessions spread through the day, such as 10 minutes in the morning, 10 minutes at lunchtime, and 10 minutes in the evening. At the end of eight weeks, both groups of engineers had improved their health and fitness profiles, and without a major difference between the groups. All had wound up with a lower heart rate and better endurance when they were evaluated on a treadmill.

More about Overload

The final concept with exercise has to do with the overload principle. Overload is not a complicated idea. The word encapsulates the concept. Overload simply means that it will improve performance as the result of systematic and progressive training of sufficient frequency, intensity, and duration. You can't keep on doing the same old workout and improve physically. The body gets used to a certain level of activity with impressive rapidity. So you have to ratchet things up.

You've no doubt experienced overload in action. Maybe you used to puff and struggle on the elliptical machine after twenty minutes and soon felt obliged to quit for the day. Then after a few weeks, those same twenty minutes became easy. From then on, you could, if you chose to, repeat that same undemanding workout (with unchanged time, distance, and resistance level) for the rest of your life and continue to maintain health benefits.

But if you wanted to become fitter, faster, or in general tougher, you had to recalibrate the resistance or prolong the workout. You would then struggle again, but you would slowly grow used to the new workout. You would have overloaded your cardiovascular and other systems, let them readjust, and from the standpoint of physical fitness, you would have improved.

How does this occur? The process is fairly simple. Physiologically, you can achieve overload by increasing the number of times you work out in a week, the length of time you work out, or the intensity of any given workout. If you enjoy walking and currently schedule five 30-minute walks in a week, you can lengthen each session to 35 minutes then to 40 minutes. As a general rule, to avoid injury you shouldn't increase your training volume by much more than 10 percent a week. But exercise of low intensity, such as walking, rarely results in injury in the first place.

You can also increase the intensity of the same workout, a concept that many athletes know and read as *intervals*. Intervals are typically short, sharp bouts of exercise performed at a measure of intensity as close to the maximum level as can be withstood, followed by rest. And then the sequence is repeated. This technique definitely results in overload and occasionally causes nausea among athletes.

Scientific study suggests, however, that applying versions of interval training can provide significant performance benefits even to walkers, recreational athletes, or anyone who wishes to improve athletically. This can easily take the form of "Walk a minute... Jog a minute..."

For the exercises themselves, please turn to *Chapter 9—Go On . . . Just Make It Happen!* You may also wish to check *Appendix A* so as to be sure that you keep your exercise plans and strategies well synchronized.

5

Food for Thought

Getting our nutrition
the way it should be

*And out of the ground the L*ORD *God made to spring up every tree that is pleasant to the sight and good for food. The tree of life was in the midst of the garden, and the tree of the knowledge of good and evil.*

(Genesis 2:9)

W hat you eat matters! Doctors in the USA report that up to one half of their patients come for medical help because, at the root of their difficulties, there are situations of eating too much, drinking too much, not getting enough sleep, or there are circumstances leading to unhappiness at home.[8] It is sometimes said that such patients need psychosomatic medical attention. The various types of antibiotics and the use of computerized medicine will often only address at a surface level the loss of health such patients are experiencing. To make a meaningful change, such individuals need to make their own choices.

Wrong Eating

There is a strong connection between food and health. In our modern age, much of the traditional wisdom with which earlier generations grew up is now being dismissed. Commercial food processing has exploded in its popularity. Too often people opt out of preparing nutritional meals, choosing rather to use convenience food simply because so little effort is involved in the preparation process.

We are witnessing an unprecedented change in eating habits today. The average person has a diet extraordinarily high in saturated fats, refined sugar and cereal, meat and other animal products, and commercially processed food. The diet is surprisingly low in fresh and raw fruits and vegetables. No longer do people save sweet and fatty foods for special occasions. Today, feasting happens every day and this form of overindulgence, albeit unintentional, is ushering people into a state of poor health.

In this connection, it is a paradox that nutritional deficiencies are common in the overfed. Such people eat much rich, sweet food, but fail to include nutritionally valuable foods, and therefore fail to get the nutrition that they would normally gain from eating simple staple foods. Nutritional deprivation through the over-consumption of high-priced, feast-time foods means that the diet of such people is thoroughly unbalanced. As a result, their health suffers.

Walters and Stanway have pointed out that, in the United States, three out of four people are estimated to die from preventable diet-related diseases. Experts agree that changes need to occur in what and how people eat. Often children grow up to become adults who habitually eat the kinds of things their parents gave them to eat as children.

In Chapter 1, we considered how it is that the fall

of humanity into sin brought about catastrophic results. Originally everything was declared by God to be very good. But when sin entered the world, widely ranging changes took place. Not only did people become separated from God, but the whole cosmos was affected. From this point, weeds would grow with good crops. There would be challenges in agriculture. It would become possible for people to abuse foods and beverages that they developed.

What we consume via the mouth does affect our health and wellbeing. People who find themselves living on a regimen of junk foods, or highly processed foodstuffs, are inviting poor health and disease issues in the medium to longer term. By not adopting a long-term policy on cooking and eating, they open themselves to negative issues they will regret. It is true that you really are what you eat! It is important in make sure that you eat in a healthy manner. If you eat a diet based on whole foods, thoughtfully prepared, the combination of these nutrients will do wonders for you. Most people only need good food—certainly not bad food plus pills!

Food Groups

The main components of a basic healthy diet are: proteins, fats, carbohydrates, minerals, vitamins, and fiber. Most whole foods contain many nutrients in varying proportions, so a variety of foods will provide a very good balance. To eat well and feel healthy, it is wise to choose whole, fresh, or carefully processed foods and favor those of vegetables or fruits. These food groups are here considered not in any particular order. They are made up as follows:

- The first food group is *carbohydrates and fiber*. This portion of a person's diet heightens the intake of starches and sugars, in contrast with those which are in rich grains, fruits, pulses (peas and beans), nuts, vegetables, and milk. Starch-rich foods, including whole grains, pulses, and bananas, should provide half of a person's calories. Fiber keeps the bowel healthy and provides protection against high cholesterol levels and even against certain forms of cancer.

- A second important part of the food group is that of *fats*. Fats provide insulation, build cells, and facilitate the metabolism. They are made of saturated, polyunsaturated, and monounsaturated fatty acid. A variety of foods provide a good balance of these.

- The third important group consists of *proteins*. Proteins contain amino acids and are used to build and repair cells and regulate one's metabolism. All fruits and vegetables contain some protein. Good sources are peas, beans, lentils, grains, nuts, seeds, sprouted seeds, and potatoes. Animal proteins are milk, cheese, meat, eggs, and fish.

- *Minerals* are another non-energy-yielding nutrient. Minerals build and maintain bones and teeth, control the composition of body fluids and cells, and release energy.

- *Vitamins* are vital for normal body chemistry. They should all come from food. Too often, people want to take supplementary pills instead of eating properly.

- Finally, *water*: water is essential to the whole system and its functions.

Getting Your Diet Right

A diet is simply a way of eating. In this respect, everyone is on a diet. People have chosen what type of food and lifestyle they are going to consistently participate in, so, whether they wake up and drink juices or whether they wake up and drink sixteen ounces of an energy drink, they are both beginning their diet for the day. That is why it is so important to take a long-term approach and decide what is best for the body. As has been mentioned before, because our bodies are the temple of the Holy Spirit—if we are believers—we must be mindful of what is going into that temple for it to be most fit for the Master's use.

It is therefore going to be important to consider what consists of a well balanced diet. Most people today eat too much fat, especially the saturated kind, and therefore that is likely to eventually add to their health problems. So it is important to cut down saturated fat intake as well as consistently watching how much fat is consumed overall. Reducing fat intake is often hard. One should concentrate on being sure that saturated fat is at a minimum; this comes from meat, poultry, eggs, milk, cheese, and butter. It is unusual for anyone to eat too much unsaturated fat. This is found in many vegetable oils and soft margarines, fatty fish, nuts, seeds, as well as in smaller amounts wholegrain cereals and some vegetables and legumes.

A very simple eating plan is as follows. You can tailor this to your own lifestyle and values.

- First, eat plenty of fiber. Whole grains, fruits, and

vegetables give you plenty of fiber as well as being associated with essential fatty acids, minerals, and vitamins.

- Secondly, eat plenty of fresh fruits and vegetables, especially green leafy ones. These give you the vitamins, minerals, essential fatty acids, and include some of the fiber you need. Peel fruit as little as possible as the peel and pith are rich in nutrients. Be sure to cook vegetables lightly by steaming or stir-frying them, and eat some of them uncooked every day, as you will benefit from their nutritional value.

- Cut down your fat intake. One way to help this is to choose fish, game, poultry, whole grains, pulses, nuts and seeds, rather than red meat and cheese.

- Cut down your sugar intake. Use sugar as flavoring rather than as a food. Limit your intake of cakes, sweets, chocolates, biscuits, puddings, ice cream, jam, fruits, soft drinks, coffee, and milkshakes. You can enjoy these, but in moderation.

- Cut down your salt intake. Instead of adding salt to your food you can accomplish much of the same by using herbs, spices, and other flavorings.

There is nothing wrong with salt in and of itself but being cautious of how much is used is beneficial.

- Reduce your consumption of processed food. Especially, avoid the "empty calories" of saturated fats, added sugar, and refined cereal grains.
- It is extremely important to drink plenty of fluids. Most people need to drink a minimum of 64 ounces of water a day. However an easy formula to remember is to drink half of your body weight in ounces of water. For example if you weigh 150 pounds, then you should drink half of the value 150, that is, 75 ounces of water daily.

Top Tips

A few simple suggestions may help. Consider the following key guidelines:

- Avoid buying high-fat, processed foods.
- Prepare food wisely.
- Be sure to check you are having adequate vitamin intake. A variety of whole grains, yellow, green, and orange fruits and vegetables, green leafy vegetables, peas and beans, nuts and seeds, fatty fish, and limited amounts of dairy and eggs, gives you a diet rich in vitamins.

- Be a more creative cook by being careful not to overindulge in salt or sugar.
- Remember that one easy way to be sure you feel full (yet without eating as much fat) is to make sure that each day you are eating three vegetable portions of food and five fruits. Eat a variety of colors.
- Cut down your fat intake. This means animal fats in the form of butter, margarine, fat and meat, whole milk, cheese, cream, and any foods made with these ingredients. When preparing foods, use vegetable oils and fats sparingly.
- Eat fish or poultry instead of red meat. These foods are lower in calories, and easier on your digestive system.
- Cut down on added sugar. This means white, brown, and multicolored sugar, as well as any foods high in sugar content.
- Reduce your intake of refined carbohydrates, including non-wholegrain breads, white breads and bagels, and foods containing refined cereal flour. Check the ingredients listed on the labels of processed foods.
- Be sure to eat high-fiber foods such as wholegrain bread, cereal, brown rice, nuts, seeds, pulses,

beans and peas, and fruits. Eating high-fiber foods helps fill you up, without adding too many calories. Eat slowly, and consider eating six small meals per day.

In the following chapter, you will find out more about the digestive system, and how to combine the various elements of nutrition when considering fats, vitamins, minerals, etc., and arranging them in a balanced diet.

6

Digest This!

Considering what happens to your food
after you have swallowed it

"Food is meant for the stomach and the stomach for food"—and God will destroy both one and the other. The body is not meant for sexual immorality, but for the Lord, and the Lord for the body.

(1 Corinthians 6:13)

Everyone eats and expends energy. Nutrition focuses on how food affects the body. It is through the science of nutrition that the digestive process comes into play. The psalmist makes the point that we are fearfully and wonderfully made (see Psalm 139:14), our inward parts having been knitted together in the wombs of our mothers (verse 13). The wonderful complexity of design reflects the brilliance of God's creative genius, and so we do well to consider how what we eat affects us.

The digestive system operates by taking whole foods and breaking them down into their chemical components. Digestion begins in the mouth and ends some twenty-seven feet later at the rectum. In the process, the body is nourished and strengthened. Whenever we swallow something, our digestive system takes care of it on autopilot. Because we are not in control of most of the digestive processes, it is easy to overlook how much work our body does.

As God has created us so intricately, and as biology books explain in detail for us, digestion begins in the mouth. When you take a bite of food, your teeth and tongue begin to mechanically break it down into smaller units. Saliva not only bathes your food with moisture, but it also allows you to taste because your taste buds work only when moisture is present. When the food has been reduced to a soft, moist mass called a bolus, your tongue pushes it to the back of your mouth and into the pharynx, where it is swallowed. After you swallow, the rest of the digestive process is involuntary. For the next two or three seconds, your food is powered by muscular contractions called peristalsis. So the bolus travels down your esophagus to your stomach.

A circular muscle called the esophageal sphincter separates the esophagus and the stomach. When you swallow, this muscle relaxes, forming an opening through which the food can pass. The rest of the time it is closed, to keep the food from moving in the opposite direction. The stomach, contrary to popular belief, is not behind the navel but higher up, in fact just below the diaphragm. This sack-like structure is shaped like the letter "J" when empty and like a boxing glove when full and food is present. The stomach expands and contracts about three times per minute to churn the food into gastric juices. These fluids, secreted by thousands of glands in the stomach lining, can consist of water, hydrochloric acid, and an enzyme called pepsin.

About one hour after a meal, the food that has been processed by the stomach, called chyme, begins to pass a little bit at a time through the pyloric sphincter into the duodenum, which is the first section of the small intestine. Most digestion and absorption occurs in the small intestine. This narrow, twisting tube, about one inch in diameter and 20 feet long, fills most of the lower abdomen. For three to six hours, peristalsis mixes and shifts the chyme through the other two sections, the jejunum and the ileum. The liver secretes bile and the pancreas secretes pancreatic enzymes into the small intestine. Bile breaks down large fat globules into small ones; pancreatic enzymes break down sugar and starch into simple sugars, fat into fatty acids, and protein into amino acids. Additional glands in the intestinal walls seek the other enzymes that break down nutrients as well. In this form, they can be absorbed. The small intestine's capacity for absorption is greatly increased by millions of tiny fingerlike projections called villi, which line its walls.

Each villus is covered by even tinier microvilli. One square inch of a small intestine contains some 20,000 villi and 10 billion microvilli. They dramatically increase the surface area of the small intestine. As a matter of fact, if you were to flatten out the small intestine completely, it would be roughly the size of a tennis court! Beneath the villis' single layer of cells are capillaries, containing simple sugars and amino acids that flow into the bloodstream, and fatty acids that enter the lymphatic system. What remains unabsorbed passes through, again by peristalsis, to the large intestine, where it spends the next 12 to 24 hours. The large intestine, about 2.5 inches in diameter and 5 to 6 feet long, is shaped like an inverted "U". It absorbs water and dissolved salts from the small intestine's residue, and its bacteria promote the breakdown of undigested materials. What remains is moved toward the rectum, the final 6 to 8 inches of the eliminating canal. The rectum stores feces until elimination.

As one can note from the digestive system, it is extremely important to have the right foods to ingest. Foods, of course, are made up of nutrients. Nutrients are substances the body can use for growth, maintenance, and repair. The body needs to take in about 43 different nutrients to function properly. Nutrients can be grouped into six categories: carbohydrates, proteins, lipids (a constituent of fat), water, vitamins, and minerals.

Energy Nutrients

The energy nutrients are carbohydrates, proteins, and fats; the non-energy nutrients are water, vitamins, and minerals. The digestive process ensures that these various nutritional components are efficiently taken into a person's bodily system and enable him to live well and to function efficiently.

Carbohydrates: The first of the six nutrients is carbohydrate. Carbohydrate is fuel for the body and brain. Carbohydrate comes in three types: simple carbohydrate, complex carbohydrate, and fiber. The U.S. Department of Agriculture (USDA), along with the U.S. Department of Health and Human Services (USDHHS), recommends that 45 to 65 percent of the total caloric intake should come from carbohydrate, which means at least 130 grams of carbohydrate per day. This minimum is required to supply the brain with an adequate amount of glucose. According to these two institutions, an adequate intake of fiber is 14 grams for every thousand calories.

Protein: The second nutrient is protein. Nothing can match protein's power for physical growth and repair. Protein is made up of amino acids, which are themselves the building blocks of cell membranes, muscle tissues, and enzymes. Although protein contains 4 calories per gram, protein is not usually a major source of energy, as rarely does it contribute more than 10 percent of daily caloric expenditure. Most Americans get between 14 and 18 percent of their calories from protein, thus falling well within the range of the 10 to 35 percent recommended by the USDHSS and USDA.

Fat: The third important nutrient is fat. Contrary to popular belief, fat is a vital ingredient in a healthy diet. Besides being the most energy-rich nutrient, fat is needed to transport vitamins, conduct nerve impulses efficiently, and cushion vital organs. It also serves as a thermal regulator and makes up a large portion of bone marrow and brain tissue. People like fat because it enhances the flavor of their food. The average American consumes between 20 to 35 percent of calories from fat.

Vitamins: The fourth nutrient is vitamins. Vitamins are critical to blood coagulation and the production of energy, hormones, enzymes, and antibodies.

Minerals: Minerals are the fifth nutrient and, in many ways, are the most important consideration when it comes to health. The body needs more than 5 grams a day of the main trace minerals, which include sodium, potassium, calcium, phosphorous, magnesium, sulfur, and chlorine. The body needs less than 5 grams per day of iron, iodine, copper, fluoride, and zinc

Water: Although water supplies no energy, vitamins or minerals, it is the most important nutrient in the body. Despite its lack of actual nutritional value, water is necessary for the excretion of vitamins, minerals, and nutrients in the food. It is also used for energy production, temperature regulation, and waste elimination. It lubricates joints, helps with digestion, and contributes to sweat production. The body's composition is 50 to 70 percent water. Muscle contains a higher concentration of water than many other tissues do—in fact, around 70 percent.

Keeping Your Diet in Balance

The U.S. Department of Agriculture (USDA) has a website that anyone can go to in order to access and track the various food groups and how much of each should be eaten. This website is www.nutrition.gov. It is possible to identify specific foods, to plan meals, and to track the nutritional values by way of an outcome.

One additional helpful website is this one, www.dietaryguidelines.gov. This will assist you not only in knowing the nutritional guidelines, but also recommended means by which you may be sure to ingest the various food groups.

7

Rest, Relaxation, and Sleep

Improving our efficiencies through wise sleep strategies

*It is in vain that you rise up early
and go late to rest,
eating the bread of anxious toil;
for he gives to his beloved sleep.*

(Psalm 127:2)

A ny recipe for a healthy lifestyle must include at least three elements: exercise, diet, and rest. Much has already been discussed about the first two. There are many books written on diet alone. Yet relatively little has been written about rest, recovery, or sleep.

In establishing a pattern or rhythm for work, God determined day and night, working week and Sabbath (Sabbath simply means "rest"), and periodic holy-days (that's where our term "holidays" comes from) at intervals throughout the year. These all enhanced the work-life balance of the people of the Old Testament, and we do well to take these principles and apply them with practical wisdom.

Circadian Rhythms[9]

Though your body rests, your brain does not. During the time you sleep, your brain prepares you for mental alertness and peak functioning the next day, especially during the rapid eye movement phase of sleep.

The need for sleep is biologically encoded. Although children need more sleep than adults, however much sleep any individual needs is genetically determined. Most adults need around eight hours of sleep per night to function at their best. You can teach yourself to sleep less but not to need less sleep.

People usually don't feel tired when they are active, but when they take a break from activity or feel bored, they may notice that they feel sleepy. The main cause of sleepiness is sleep deprivation. Boredom doesn't cause sleepiness, but it does reveal it.

Sleep is as necessary to your health as food and water are, and rest is no substitute for it. When you don't get the sleep you need, your body builds up a sleep debt that can only be repaid with sleep.

Most people don't remember their dreams, but everyone does dream every night. Dreams are most vivid during the rapid eye movement phase of sleep, which is the deepest sleep that people achieve. The need for sleep remains constant throughout adulthood. Older people often awaken more frequently and sleep less during the night but they tend to make up for that during the day through occasional napping. Sleep difficulties are not an inevitable part of aging, although they are, in fact, very common.

Human beings, like all other living things, have circadian rhythms that affect when they feel alert and when they feel sleepy. Circadian rhythms are set by the cycle of daylight. During travel across time zones, your body quickly adjusts because the cycle changes, but when you work a night shift, your body never adjusts because the cycle does not change.

Sleep disorders must be treated. Unfortunately, many people who have them don't realize they are problems that can be treated. Untreated sleep disorders can ruin your quality of life, your performance at work, and your relationships with other people.

Good Night!

It is amazing how important sleep is to any individual. The following are some very practical ideas to help you achieve good sleep and to gain the benefits from it. Before reading the list, keep in mind that it is not a good practice to eat just before you go to bed, as your body then has to work on the process of digesting when, in fact, it should be resting!

Establish a consistent sleep schedule. Go to bed and wake up at the same time 365 days a year. Many experts believe that after getting enough sleep, this is the most important thing you can do to wake up feeling refreshed. One of the most important aspects of a consistent sleep schedule is to make it a priority.

You'll find what works best for you. Some people like to go to bed early and wake up early. Some like to go to bed later and wake up later. The ultimate test of adequate sleep is that you do not need to wake up to an alarm clock. To really be serious about this, you may need to force yourself to go to bed earlier and earlier each evening so that eventually you are waking up without an alarm clock. If you find that you need a short nap during the days of adjustment when you are getting accustomed to adequate sleep, a power nap—that is a short nap of seven to twelve minutes—will do wonders in helping you get back on schedule.

Get regular exercise. Exercise also helps people sleep well. You may need to be sure of the time frame you are exercising in. If you exercise too late in the day or evening, it may act as a stimulant which then wakens you. Again, as with your sleeping pattern, find what works best for you in the overall scheme of things.

Consider establishing a bedtime ritual. Allowing yourself to stay up late at night watching TV so that you fall asleep is not a good ritual. It is better to go to your bed and read or pray and meditate, or listen to soothing music. The routine must be regular and consistent to be effective. Many people recommend using your bed only for sleep. Doing work, talking on the phone, or watching TV in bed may send conflicting messages to your brain about what should happen there.

Create a quality sleeping environment. This may include factors such as quietness, darkness, and ambient temperature. Some people are able to go to sleep right away. Others may need to have music or a low level of white noise (such as made by a fan) to fall asleep. Whatever it takes, find what works for you. You may need to take practical steps to make your room dark by getting opaque blinds for your windows, turning off your computer screen and other electronic devices, turning digital clocks away from you, and positioning a towel against the door to limit light seeping in from the hallways. If these measures are not enough, you can purchase special blinds to block out light.

Invest in a quality bed and sleeping accessories. Most people spend almost a third of their lives in bed, so making a comfortable bed is worth the investment.

When you are considering the size of the bed, make sure it is big enough. Also make sure that your sheets are comfortable, easy to care for, and durable. Be sure you have a pillow that is comfortable and suitable for your own needs.

Be aware of conditions such as sleep apnea. Although somewhat uncommon, sleep apnea is a condition that some people have and are not aware of. Diagnosis is usually done in a sleeping clinic where the patient is monitored electronically through the night. People who have been diagnosed with sleep apnea generally respond very well to therapy, and most patients report dramatic recovery of health and energy once this condition has been addressed.

8

Blessed Are the Balanced!

Maintaining body-soul equilibrium

I appeal to you therefore, brothers, by the mercies of God, to present your bodies as a living sacrifice, holy and acceptable to God, which is your spiritual worship.

(Romans 12:1)

There are always going to be ideas on how to lose weight. A weight-reducing diet may be necessary for a time, but for the long haul, you need to make sure that what you eat is consistently a natural part of your lifestyle, and therefore one that ensures your weight remains relatively constant.

An Apple a Day Keeps the Dietician Away!

One idea for a healthy way to feel full (and it's one which may assist you in both feeling healthy and losing weight) is simply to eat an apple before you eat anything else. By eating an apple before each meal, you will fill up and not need to eat as much other food in your meal. Eating an apple in this way will help provide your fruit as well as roughage for the day. If you repeat this procedure three, four, or five times during the day, it will work wonders in controlling your feelings of hunger and reducing the amount of fat that you consume.

Another very important aspect of losing weight is to be sure you are drinking the amount of water that is necessary for your weight. This was previously discussed as drinking half of the value of your body's weight (measured in pounds but expressed in ounces) in water.[10]

If you have decided that you want to lose weight, you may be tempted to hurry up the weight-loss process. It is important to decide ultimately how much weight you would like to lose and then spread that over a period of six months to one year. By doing that, depending on your weight loss goal, it will allow you to lose between a quarter of a pound to a half a pound a week. The number of calories that you will need to reduce for this will be quite minimal. By taking a long-range view on this, you will find it will do wonders in making it so much easier to lose that weight. Too often, people will go on a "crash" diet, meaning they drastically reduce their food intake, which will initially help them lose weight rapidly and which, for a time, will be very encouraging. However, rapidly reducing their food intake is not sustainable and they will usually be back on their original diet of overeating before they know it. Yo-yo dieting can wreak havoc with a person's metabolism (this kind of crash dieting forces the body into starvation mode and the body holds on to its fat) so the net result is often an overall weight gain.

There are many electronic applications available to help keep track of your eating.[11] Just noting or recording what you eat and how much is consumed may be all it takes to get you into a healthy or healthier eating plan.

One way of doing this is to initially record your body weight, and then, on your dietary program, you should formulate your goal weight. With these simple steps in place, such electronic applications can calculate out how long it will take you to lose weight. By consistently following this simple weight-loss strategy, you will be helped to reduce weight, and by doing this over a long period of time, you will develop the good habits of a healthy eating style.

Another very important aspect of losing weight, and eventually (or consistently) maintaining your weight, is through exercise. A person consumes calories so as to get enough energy to function throughout the day. When an individual burns these calories through exercise, it actually allows him or her to consume more calories each day because many more calories are being burned. So, an easy formula for weight loss is to be sure that you take in fewer calories than you burn.

When people initially set out to do this and begin writing down what they eat, they realize without any doubt how much they are consuming. After initially understanding how much food is being consumed, when they formulate a goal, they will find it so much easier to reduce overall caloric consumption.[12]

As tempting as it may be to try a fad diet, an infomercial, or a celebrity-endorsed diet, it is best to avoid such. If you happen to go off your diet for a day or more, do not give up. It is the long haul that counts. Be gentle and forgiving with yourself and go back to the diet as soon as you can. If you happen to overeat as part of your comfort and reward system, think of an alternative or a substitute for this. Sometimes when a person is looking for comfort or a reward, it is better to do something active rather than to eat something that is tasty. A craving for food may be brought on by either a lack of hydration or a deficiency in rest. That is why it is so important to lead a balanced and holistic life. Food intake, along with adequate exercise, will help to maintain a proper body weight.

Quench That Thirst!

Did you know that a lack of hydration can even cause quite intense headaches? A common rule to remember is this: Drink water before you are thirsty! If you are unwell, or experiencing hydration loss through a gastric episode—or even if you have spent extra time outdoors in warm weather—you may well have lost liquid that you are not aware of, and a headache is the outcome. Be sure to monitor your liquid intake under such circumstances. And there is nothing to beat old-fashioned water!

Speaking in Spiritual Terms ...

For Christians, it is so important to keep in mind the reality of their bodies being temples of the Holy Spirit (1 Corinthians 6:19). If you are a believer, you are not your own; you have been purchased with a price, and therefore you are to glorify God in your body. The apostle Paul wrote in Philippians 3:19 that believers are not to allow their bellies to be their god! It has been said that we are to eat to live, not that we live to eat!

Thankfully, God is near to us when we call upon Him! He never places more responsibilities upon us than those which can be completely managed. 1 Corinthians 10:13 clearly teaches that there is "no temptation" that is too great for us to bear, and we can, with God's help, overcome what seems difficult. That means that even food intake and unwise consumption can be avoided. In James 1:2-4 we read that, when difficulties come—and this can include even matters such as challenges in our eating—we can count it all joy, for such trials produce steadfastness, which, in turn, help us to be complete for God's glory. While unwise eating may be a huge temptation to some, the matter can be overcome through considering it as a trial, and asking God to help.

Understanding that God cares about the whole you—your body as much as your soul—may be a new starting point for you. You honor God when you care for your body and soul. God loves and cares for all of you! What happens in your body is not unrelated to the soul-spirit aspect that makes up the total you.

Understanding these things serves as a strong motivation to respond to the call of Romans 12:1. Because of God's mercies to us in the gospel—because of a Savior who Himself purchased redemption for us by offering up His own body as a sacrifice—is it really too much for us to respond in glad and willing obedience to offer up our own bodies to Him in practical and careful service as living sacrifices? Christ is not only the Savior of our souls, but the Savior of our bodies. There is yet a time to come when our mortal bodies shall be redeemed, and in the final state, we shall have resurrected, glorified bodies in which to live (see 1 Corinthians 15)!

9

Go On . . . Just Make It Happen!

Putting the principles into practice

How long will you lie there, O sluggard?
When will you arise from your sleep?
A little sleep, a little slumber,
a little folding of the hands to rest,
and poverty will come upon you like a robber,
and want like an armed man.

Proverbs 6:9-11

What more needs to be said? All you have to do now is to turn the page and review the exercises you plan to use. Use the charts in the appendix sections to help you plan and regulate your exercises.

So now that you have decided to embark on your journey of fitness, or continue where you have left off, please know, that as God has said in His Word, "You will reap what you sow" (see Galatians 6:7)! In other words, as you begin to slowly improve your fitness, you will realize that your efforts are paying off. You will be able to enjoy not only the result of your efforts, but the process as well! As you exercise, you will enjoy the benefits of good rest, fewer hours of sleep needed, more efficient processing of foods, and an overall better feeling as your endorphins are continually released!

On your mark... get set... get fit!

1 BACK / LEG STRETCHES

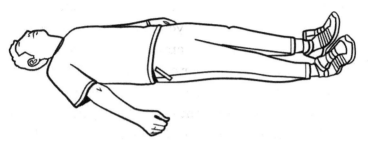

Figure 1(a): Relaxed position: Lie down on back with arms
outstretched and legs straight ahead.

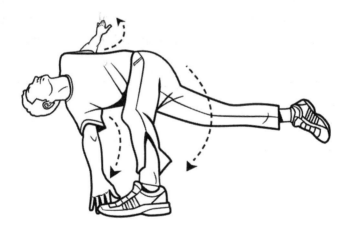

Figure 1(b): Retracted position: Lift left leg, and stretch it across
the body, trying to touch the right hand. Hold for 30 seconds.
Repeat with the opposite leg.

107

2 HAMSTRING STRETCHES

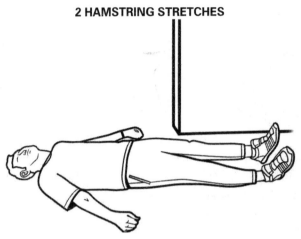

Figure 2(a): Relaxed position: Lie down on back with legs next to secure object.

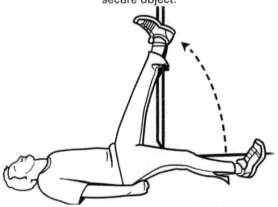

Figure 2(b): Retracted position: Lift left leg, and place against the secure object, stretching the hamstring. Hold for 30 seconds. Repeat with the opposite leg.

3 IT BAND STRETCHES

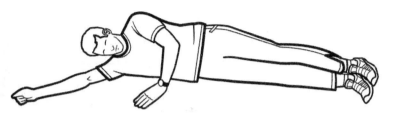

Figure 3(a): Relaxed position: Lie down on side with right arm outstretched and legs stretched out and together.

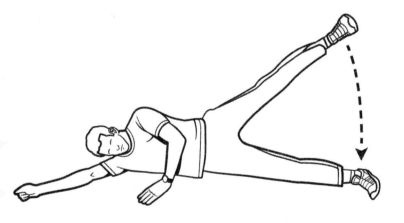

Figure 3(b): Retracted position: While right arm is outstretched, raise left leg and return to relaxed position, and repeat 30 times. Repeat on opposite side.

4 PUSH UPS

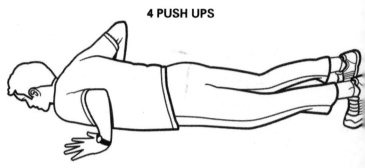

Figure 4(a): Relaxed position: Lie flat on your stomach. Start with as many repetitions as feels comfortable. Set your own goal, and increase to that completion.

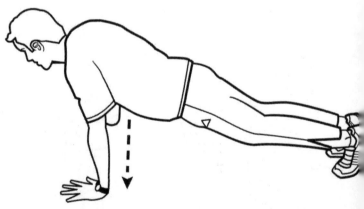

Figure 4(b): Retracted position: Extend arms so that torso and legs raise up, then lower. Start with 3 repetitions, and work up to being able to doing 30 at one time.

110

5 HAMSTRING / CALF STRETCHES

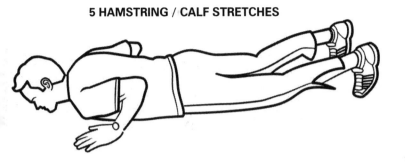

Figure 5(a): Relaxed position: Lie down on stomach with arms by side.

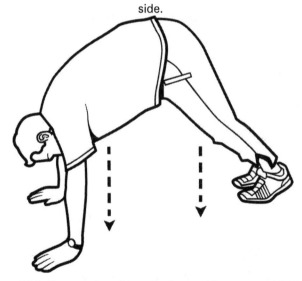

Figure 5(b): Retracted position: Push up with arms, and lift torso and buttocks high in the air so hamstrings and calves are stretched. Hold for 30 seconds.

111

6 GROIN STRETCHES

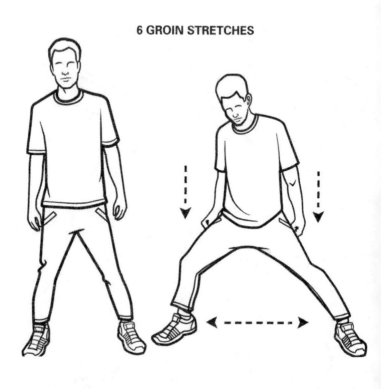

Figure 6(a): Relaxed position: Stand with legs at shoulder width and arms hanging loosely.

Figure 6(b): Retracted position: Lift left leg, and step a distance to put a stretch on the inner thigh muscle. Hold this stretch for 30 seconds. Repeat with the opposite leg.

7 QUAD STRETCHES

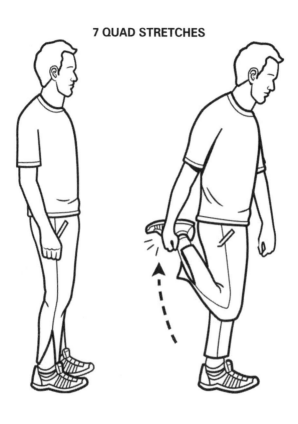

Figure 7(a): Relaxed position: Stand with both legs straight.

Figure 7(b): Retracted position: Lift right leg, bending at the knee, and hold right foot with right hand for 30 seconds. Repeat with other leg.

8 PLANK COMPREHENSIVE

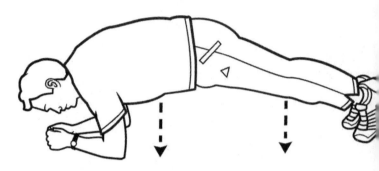

Figure 8(a): Retracted: On stomach, raise torso and place body weight on elbows, keeping legs straight. Hold for 30 seconds.

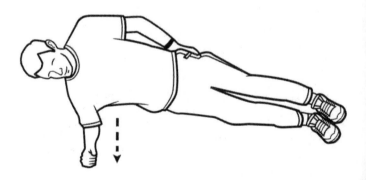

Figure 8(b): Retracted: Keep same position as stomach retracted, roll to elbow, keeping legs straight and weight on one elbow and hold for 30 seconds.

8 PLANK COMPREHENSIVE

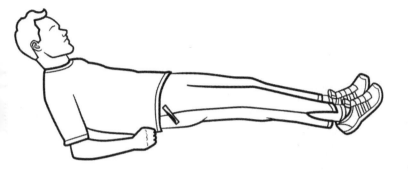

Figure 8(c): Keep in same position as 8(b); roll to back, with weight on elbows, keeping legs straight. Hold for 30 seconds.

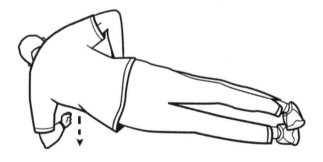

Figure 8(d): Retracted position: Roll on to opposite elbow as 8(b) and follow exact instructions from 10 (b) and hold for 30 seconds.

115

9 LUNGES

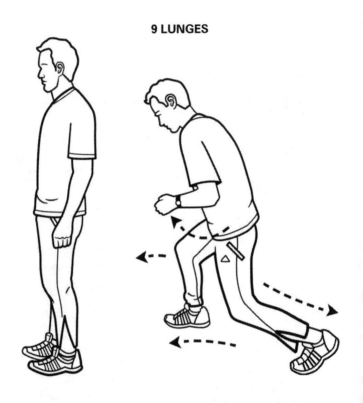

Figure 9(a): Relaxed position: stand with both legs straight.

Figure 9(b): Retracted position: Extend right leg as far as possible, then bend left knee, and hold for 30 seconds. Repeat on opposite side.

10 PULL UPS

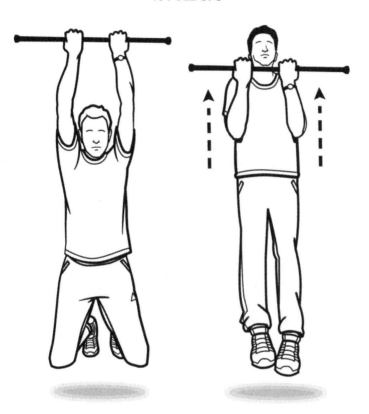

Figure 10(a): Relaxed position: Hang from a secure bar.

Figure 10(b): Retracted position: Pull up with arms so that chin raises above the bar, and return to relaxed position. Start with what you feel comfortable with, set goal, and work to completion.

117

11 ABDOMINAL CRUNCHES

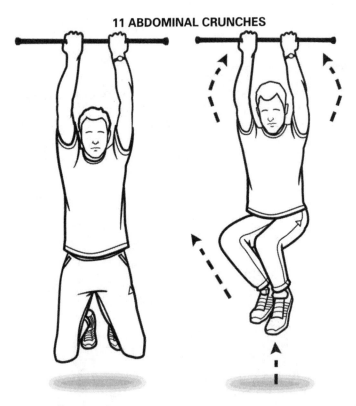

Figure 11(a): Relaxed position: Hang from same bar used for pull up.

Figure 11(b): Retracted position: Raise knees up to stomach for abdominal crunch. Raise knees as far left as possible, and then repeat on other side, for oblique crunch. Start with as many repetitions as feels comfortable. Set your own goal, and increase to that completion.

12 MEDICINE BALL SIT UPS

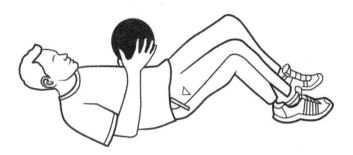

Figure 12(a): Relaxed position: While lying flat on back, hold medicine ball on stomach.

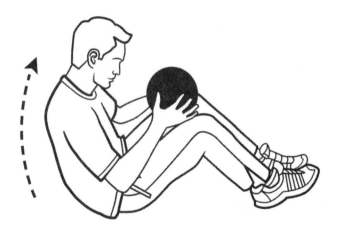

Figure 12(b): Retracted position: Sit up with the ball and touch your knees, and then return. Repeat for 30 seconds.

13 MEDICINE BALL SQUATS

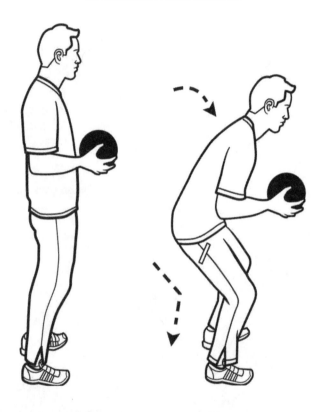

Figure 13(a): Relaxed position: Hold a medicine ball at waist.

Figure 13(b): Retracted position: Bend knees to 45 degrees and then return. Repeat as many times as you can in 30 seconds. Repeat on other side.

14 DUMB BELLS

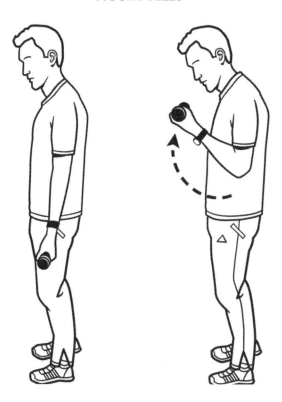

Figure 14(a): Relaxed position: Hold a dumbbell in each hand at waist.

Figure 14(b): Retracted position: Raise dumbbells, alternating left and right arm, for 30 seconds.

15 SIT UPS

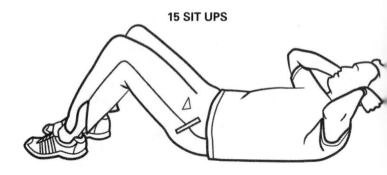

Figure 15(a): Relaxed position: Lie flat on your back. Start with as many repetitions as feels comfortable. Set your own goal, and increase to that completion.

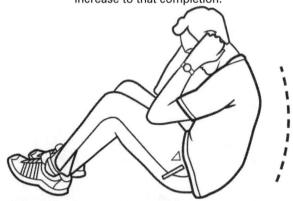

Figure 15(b): Retracted position: Leave fists at ear level, and having knees bent, raise so that elbows touch knees, and return. Start with 3 repetitions, and work up to being able to do 30 at one time.

Appendix A

Exercise Charts

The charts on the following pages will help you to plan and regulate your exercise routine in a systematic and disciplined manner.

You may download copies of these charts for your own use (and only your use) from the following website: www.fitforthemaster.fit

MILEAGE BUILD UP (2 MILES)

Week	Day One	Day Two	Day Three
Week One	W-.5, R-.25, W-.25	W-.5, R-.25, W-.25	W-.25, R-.5, W-.25
Week Two	W-.5, R-.5, W-.25	W-.5, R-.5, W-.25	W-.25, R-.5, W-.5
Week Three	W-.25, R-.75, W-.25	W-.5, R-.5, W-.5	W-.25, R-.75, W-.5
Week Four	W-.5, R-.5, W-.5	W-.5, R-.5, W-.5	W-.25, R.-.75, W-.75
Week Five	W-.5, R-1, W-.25	W-.75, R-.75, W-.5	W-.5, R-1, W-.5
Week Six	W.25, R-1.25, W-.25	W-.5, R-.1, W-.5	W-.25, R-1.5, W-.25
Week Seven	W.-25, R-1.5, W-.25	W.-.5, R-.1.25, W-.25	W-.25, R-1.75
Week Eight	W-.25, R-1.75	W-.25, R-1.75	R-2

MILEAGE BUILD UP (2 MILES) EXPLANATION

W=Walk (Walk with the same stride—don't speed up and slow down—maintain a level pace.)

R=Run (Run—make sure you pace yourself so that you maintain the same stride length and speed the entire run.)

.25=One-quarter mile (one lap around track)

.5=Half mile (two laps around track)

.75=Three-quarter mile (three laps around track)

1=Full mile (four laps around track)

Don't settle for what you haven't been able to do in the past.

Use this as a goal, not only for two miles, but you can use the same ratio and work up to five miles.

Using this same ratio can be used for biking and swimming as well.

WEEKLY RUNNING CHART: (5K)

Week	M	T	W	TH	F	S
One	2	2 S	3	2 T	R	3
Two	?	2 S	2.5	2 T	R	3
Three	3	3 S	2	2 T	R	3
Four	2	2.5 S	2.5	3 T	R	4
Five	2	3 S	3	3 T	R	4
Six	3	2 S	4	2 T	R	4
Seven	3	3 S	2	2 T	R	4
Eight	3	2 S	4	3 T	R	5
Nine	4	3 S	2	R	R	5
Ten	3	3 S	R	3 T	3	6
Eleven	3	2 S	2 S	2 T	3	3
Twelve	2	3 S	2	R	R	5 K

WEEKLY RUNNING EXPLANATIONS (5K)

The numbers listed are for miles to be run, and are to be run at conversational speed–can talk while running.

S=Run your distance, but within the distance stated, pick a point ahead of you 100 yards or so, and "stride" at a quicker pace than normal to that spot, and then keep running, don't stop, at your regular pace. "Stride" every 5 minutes of your run.

T=Run your distance, but within your distance, run 1.5 - 2.0 miles at a "tempo" faster than conversational speed, or run that tempo for 12 - 16 minutes.

R=Rest–no running, but may cross train if wanted.

WEEKLY RUNNING CHART (10K)

Week	M	T	W	TH	F	S
One	2	2 S	3	2 T	R	3
Two	3	3 S	3	3 T	R	4
Three	3	3 S	3	3 T	R	4
Four	2	4 S	4	4 T	R	4
Five	2	4 S	3	3 T	R	5
Six	3	3 S	4	2 T	R	5
Seven	4	4 S	4	4 T	R	5
Eight	4	3 S	4	3 T	R	6
Nine	4	3 S	2	R	R	6
Ten	3	4 S	R	4 T	3	6
Eleven	3	3 S	R	3 T	3	3
Twelve	4	3 S	2	R	R	10 K

WEEKLY RUNNING EXPLANATION (10K)

The numbers listed are for miles to be run, and are to be run at conversational speed–can talk while running.

S=Run your distance, but within the distance stated, pick a point ahead of you 100 yds or so, and "stride" at a quicker pace than normal to that spot, and then keep running, don't stop, at your regular pace. "Stride" every 5 minutes of your run.

T=Run your distance, but within your distance, run 1.5 - 2.0 miles at a "tempo" faster than conversational speed, or run that tempo for 12 - 16 minutes.

R=Rest–no running, but may cross train if wanted.

HALF-MARATHON RUNNING SCHEDULE

Week	M	T	W	TH	F	S
One	2	2 S	3	R	R	3
Two	3	R	3	3 T	R	4
Three	3	3 S	3	R	R	4
Four	2	4 S	4	R	R	4
Five	2	R	3	3 T	R	5
Six	3	R	4	2 T	R	5
Seven	4	4 S	4	R	R	5
Eight	4	R	4	3 T	R	6
Nine	4	3 S	2	R	R	6
Ten	3	4 S	R	4 T	3	6
Eleven	3	3 S	R	3 T	3	3
Twelve	4	3 S	2	R	R	6
Thirteen	4	4 S	R	4 T	R	7
Fourteen	5	5 S	R	5 T	R	8
Fifteen	5	5 S	5	R	R	10
Sixteen	5	5 S	5	5 T	R	5
Sev'teen	5	5 S	5	5 T	R	10
Eighteen	4	5 S	5	5 T	R	8
Nineteen	3	3	5	5	R	6
Twenty	2	2	R	R	R	Half M'th

HALF-MARATHON RUNNING SCHEDULE EXPLANATION

The numbers listed are for miles to be run, and are to be run at conversational speed–can talk while running.

S=Run your distance, but within the distance stated, pick a point ahead of you 100 yds or so, and "stride" at a quicker pace than normal to that spot, then maintain regular pace. "Stride" every 5 minutes of your run.

T=Run your distance, but within your distance, run 1.5 - 2.0 miles at a "tempo" faster than conversational speed, or run that tempo for 12 - 16 minutes.

R=Rest–no running, but may cross train if desired.

FULL MARATHON RUNNING SCHEDULE

Week	M	T	W	TH	F	S
One	2	2 S	3	2 T	R	5
Two	3	3 S	3	3 T	R	6
Three	3	4 S	3	4 T	R	7
Four	5	3 S	3	3 T	R	5
Five	4	4 S	3	4 T	R	8
Six	3	4 S	2	2 T	R	6
Seven	5	5 S	5	R	R	10
Eight	5	5 S	5	R	R	8
Nine	5	5 S	R	5 T	R	12
Ten	5	5 S	5	R	3	8
Eleven	3	5 S	5	5 T	R	14
Twelve	5	5 T	5	5 S	R	9
Thirteen	5	5 S	R	5 T	R	16
Fourteen	5	5 T	5	R	R	10
Fifteen	5	5 S	5	R	R	18
Sixteen	R	5	5	5	R	14
Sev'teen	5	5 S	5 T	5	R	20
Eighteen	R	5	5 S	5 T	5	12
Nin'teen	2	2	3	R	5	10
Twenty	2	2	R	R	R	Marathon

FULL MARATHON RUNNING SCHEDULE EXPLANATION

The numbers listed are for miles to be run, and are to be run at conversational speed–can talk while running.

S=Run your distance, but within the distance stated, pick a point ahead of you 100 yds or so, and "stride" at a quicker pace than normal to that spot, then maintain regular pace. "Stride" every 5 minutes of your run.

T=Run your distance, but within your distance, run 1.5 - 2.0 miles at a "tempo" faster than conversational speed., or run that tempo for 12 - 16 minutes.

R=Rest–no running, but may cross train if desired.

CENTURY TRAINING SCHEDULE (BIKING)

Week	M	T	W	TH	F	S
One	40	30 S	30	40 T	R	60
Two	50	30 S	30	60 T	R	75
Three	60	40 S	30	40 T	R	75
Four	60	50 S	45	60 T	R	90
Five	60	40 S	30	40 T	R	100
Six	75	50 S	50	50 T	R	120
Seven	75	50 S	70	60 T	R	150
Eight	75	75 S	75	75 T	R	180
Nine	75	75 S	R	75 T	R	120
Ten	90	90 S	50	90 T	R	180
Eleven	90	90 S	50	60 T	R	140
Twelve	50	50 T	50	50 S	R	90
Thirteen	90	90 S	R	90 T	R	160
Fourteen	90	75 T	60	60 T	R	200
Fifteen	100	50 S	50	90 T	R	240
Sixteen	100	100 S	100	100 T	R	140
Sev'nteen	120	120 S	50 T	R	R	300
Eighteen	R	50	50 S	50 T	50	120
Nineteen	100	120	30	R	50	120
Twenty	60	60	R	R	R	Century

CENTURY TRAINING SCHEDULE (BIKING)
EXPLANATION

The numbers listed are for time (minutes) on your bike at conversational speed–can talk while riding

S=Pick up your speed within your distance, and pick a point ahead of you 100 yds or so, and "sprint" at a quicker pace than normal to that spot, then maintain regular pace. "Sprint" every 5 minutes.

T=Pick up your speed in your distance for short bursts of 1-5 minutes at a "tempo" faster than conversational

R=Rest–no riding, but may cross train if desired.

SWIMMING: ONE-MILE BUILD UP SCHEDULE

Week	M	T	W	TH	F	S
One	50	R	50	R	75	R
Two	75	R	75	R	100	R
Three	100	R	100	R	150	R
Four	150	R	150	R	200	R
Five	200	R	200	R	275	R
Six	250	R	250	R	300	R
Seven	300	R	300	R	350	R
Eight	350	R	350	R	400	R
Nine	400	R	400	R	500	R
Ten	500	R	500	R	600	R
Eleven	575	R	575	R	700	R
Twelve	650	R	650	R	800	R
Thirteen	725	R	725	R	900	R
Fourteen	800	R	800	R	100	R
Fifteen	875	R	875	R	1100	R
Sixteen	950	R	950	R	1200	R
Sev'teen	1025	R	1125	R	1300	R
Eighteen	1125	R	1225	R	1400	R
Nineteen	1225	R	1325	R	1500	R
Twenty	800	R	800	R	1600	R

SWIMMING: ONE-MILE BUILD UP EXPLANATION

Numbers represent meters. Typically, a pool is either 25 meters in length, or 25 yards.

Some pools, Olympic distance ones, are 50 meters in length. Do the math to adjust if needs be!

R stands for recovery day, or you may cross-train on these days as well.

You may incorporate all strokes (breast, back, side, and crawl) within the work out, or you may prefer to stick to one.

CIRCUIT TRAINING SCHEDULE

Week	Day One	Day Two	Day Three
Week One	Leg Press—5; Calf Raises—5 Chest Press—5; Dead Lift—5 Shoulder Press—5; Lat Pull down—5 Ab Press—5; Back Pull—5 Aerobics—5 min.	Leg Press5; Calf Raises—5 Chest Press—5; Dead Lift—5 Shoulder Press—5; Lat Pull down—5 Ab Press—5; Back Pull—5 Aerobics—5 min.	Leg Press5; Calf Raises—5 Chest Press—5; Dead Lift—5 Shoulder Press—5; Lat Pull down—5 Ab Press—5; Back Pull—5 Aerobics—5 min.
Week Two	Leg Press—6; Calf Raises—6 Chest Press—6; Dead Lift—6 Shoulder Press—6; Lat Pull down—6 Ab Press—6; Back Pull—6 Aerobics—5 min.	Leg Press—6; Calf Raises—6 Chest Press—6; Dead Lift—6 Shoulder Press—6; Lat Pull down—6 Ab Press—6; Back Pull—6 Aerobics—5 min.	Leg Press—5; Calf Raises—5 Chest Press—5; Dead Lift—5 Shoulder Press—5; Lat Pull down—5 Ab Press—5; Back Pull—5 Aerobics—5 min.
Week Three	Leg Press—7; Calf Raises—7 Chest Press—7; Dead Lift—7 Shoulder Press—7; Lat Pull down—7 Ab Press—7; Back Pull—7 Aerobics—5 min.	Leg Press—7; Calf Raises—7 Chest Press—7; Dead Lift—7 Shoulder Press—7; Lat Pull down—7 Ab Press—7; Back Pull—7 Aerobics—5 min.	Leg Press—7; Calf Raises—7 Chest Press—7; Dead Lift—7 Shoulder Press—7; Lat Pull down—7 Ab Press—7; Back Pull—7Aerobics—5 min.

Week	Day One	Day Two	Day Three
Week Four	Leg Press—8; Calf Raises—8 Chest Press—8; Dead Lift—8 Shoulder Press—8; Lat Pull down—8 Ab Press—8; Back Pull—8 Aerobics—5 min.	Leg Press—8; Calf Raises—8 Chest Press—8; Dead Lift—8 Shoulder Press—8; Lat Pull down—8 Ab Press—8; Back Pull—8 Aerobics—5 min.	Leg Press—8; Calf Raises—8 Chest Press—8; Dead Lift—8 Shoulder Press—8; Lat Pull down—8 Ab Press—8; Back Pull—8 Aerobics—5 min.
Week Five	Leg Press—9; Calf Raises—9 Chest Press—9; Dead Lift—9 Shoulder Press—9; Lat Pull down—9 Ab Press—9; Back Pull—9 Aerobics—5 min.	Leg Press—9; Calf Raises—9 Chest Press—9; Dead Lift—9 Shoulder Press—9; Lat Pull down—9 Ab Press—9; Back Pull—9 Aerobics—5 min.	Leg Press—9; Calf Raises—9 Chest Press—9; Dead Lift—9 Shoulder Press—9; Lat Pull down—9 Ab Press—9; Back Pull—9 Aerobics—5 min.
Week Six	Leg Press—10; Calf Raises—10 Chest Press—10; Dead Lift—10 Shoulder Press—10; Lat Pull down—10 Ab Press—10; Back Pull—10 Aerobics—5 min.	Leg Press—10; Calf Raises—10 Chest Press—10; Dead Lift—10 Shoulder Press—10; Lat Pull down—10 Ab Press—10; Back Pull—10 Aerobics—5 min.	Leg Press—10; Calf Raises—10 Chest Press—10; Dead Lift—10 Shoulder Press—10; Lat Pull down—10 Ab Press—10; Back Pull—10 Aerobics—5 min.

CIRCUIT TRAINING—A FULL-BODY WORKOUT: EXPLANATION

Circuit Training—this includes lifting weights and an aerobic workout per circuit. Each circuit would encompass what is in the one cell in the chart. You may set your own resistance weight for each exercise, but use the number listed as repetitions for the specific weight. The aerobic segment can be on any piece of equipment (elliptical, treadmill, stationary bike, rowing machine). The six weeks should keep the same weight resistance per exercise, but increase the number of repetitions. After the six weeks, you may start over with a little more resistance. Seek to do three circuits per session.

In summary, note the following:

- Leg press—Exercise which strengthens the quads and hamstrings;
- Calf raises—Exercise which increases the calf muscle;
- Chest press—Exercise which strengthens the chest;
- Shoulder press—Exercise which strengthens the shoulders;
- Lat pulldown—Exercise which strengthens the neck and shoulders;
- Ab press—Exercise which strengthens the core;
- Back pull—Exercise which strengthens the back.

Appendix B

Useful Reference Resources

During the course of years, I have read and gleaned extensive information, not only from books such as the ones listed below, but from many colleagues and associates. Many of the points considered in this book are matters of general knowledge. The four books listed below have been useful sources for some of the information shared here.

- Larsen, Laura (2010). *Fitness and Exercise Sourcebook*, Detroit, MI: Omnigraphics Inc
- Lloyd-Jones, D. Martyn (1998). *Healing and the Scriptures*. Nashville, TN: Thomas Nelson
- Stanway, Penny (1989). *Foods for Common Ailments*. New York, NY: Simon & Schuster
- Walters, Peter and John Byl (2013). *Christian Paths to Health and Wellness*. Champaign, IL: Human Kinetics

For Further Reading

- Fleck, S.J. & Kraemer, W.J. (2014). *Designing resistance training programs (4th ed.).* Champaign, IL: Human Kinetics.
- Heyward, V.H. & Gibson, A.L. (2014). *Advanced fitness assessment and exercise prescription (7th ed.).* Champaign, IL: Human Kinetics.
- Howley, E.T. & Franks, B.D. (2007). *Fitness professional's handbook (5th ed.).* Champaign, IL: Human Kinetics.
- National Strength and Conditioning Association (2008). Baechle, T.R. & Earle, R.W. (Eds.). *Essentials of strength training and conditioning (3rd ed.).* Champaign, IL: Human Kinetics.
- Corbin, C.B. & LeMasurier, G.C. (2014). *Fitness for life (6th ed.).* Champaign, IL: Human Kinetics.
- Donatelle, R.J. (2015). *Health: The basics (11th ed.).* Boston: Pearson.
- Hutchinson, A. (2011). *Which comes first, cardio or weights? Fitness myths, training truths, and other surprising discoveries from the science of exercise.* New York: Harper.

Postscript

Join the Conversation!

So, you have started on this great journey back to health and wellness. Well done! Just as with everything else in life, you will find there are plenty of ups and downs. But I would love to hear your story, and to encourage you along the way.

Please connect with me. I'd love for you to visit my website, www.fitforthemaster.fit, and click on the link to join my mailing list and receive periodic updates via my blog. And please find me on Facebook at the address below—I'd love for you to become a friend!

https://www.facebook.com/john.lehman.165

Go on; join the conversation—I'd just love to hear from you!

John Lehman
www.fitforthemaster.fit

Endnotes

[1] D. Martyn Lloyd-Jones; see the details of his book in the bibliography. "The Doctor," as he was known, knew about people's souls and bodies.

[2] Peter Walters and John Byl; see details of this book in the bibliography.

[3] Laura Larsen has written helpfully in this area. See details of her book in the bibliography.

[4] These and other points are suggested by Laura Larsen.

[5] I am indebted to my friend Dr. Brent Heidorn for this acronym.

[6] For a specific scenario of how this may be applied, refer to Chapter 3.

[7] Penny Stanway; her book is referenced in the bibliography.

[8] Penny Stanway; see above.

[9] *Circadian* means "around the day," that is, at approximately twenty-four-hour intervals.

[10] See Chapter 5.

[11] See USDA website details in Chapter 5.

[12] For further information, see "Top Tips" in Chapter 5, where there are several easy-to-take steps that you may follow.